Making Babies

A Personal View of IVF

by

Lord Winston

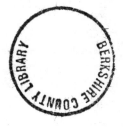

BBC BOOKS

This book is published to accompany the television series
entitled *Making Babies* which was first broadcast in 1996. The series was
produced bythe BBC Documentaries department.
Executive Producer: Olivia Lichtenstein
Producer: Joanna Clinton Davis

Published by BBC Books,
an imprint of BBC Worldwide Publishing,
BBC Worldwide Limited, Woodlands,
80 Wood Lane, London W12 0TT

First published 1996
ISBN 0 563 38721 1

Designed by Edward Moody Design Ltd

Set in Adobe Stone
Printed in Great Britain by Martins the Printers Ltd,
Bound in Great Britain by Hunter & Foulis Ltd, Edinburgh
Cover printed by Richard Clays, St Ives plc

This book is dedicated to two people who have had such a powerful influence on my thinking and who have guided me in terms of the difficult issues raised in this book.

Firstly, to Dr R.H. Ellis, my close friend and anaesthetist for twenty years, who died tragically and suddenly in 1995. Dick was a most upright gentleman and a wonderful doctor whose practice exemplified the highest medical standards. His careful and sane appraisal of these reproductive issues was invariably wise. His guidance is badly missed.

Secondly, to Dr R.A. Margara, my close friend and colleague and another true gentleman. He remains a great pillar of strength in my life. There is no doctor in the field of reproductive medicine who has higher ethical standards. His sense of service, his balance and propriety, and his advice have all been crucial in all my thinking.

Contents

Acknowledgments

I am, as always, grateful to my wife Lira, who yet again has – with her typical forbearance and gentleness – put up with my behaviour during the preparation of another book. I am indebted to Maggie Pearlstine, the best of agents, for her friendship, advice and encouragement in all aspects of my writing; and to Matthew Baylis, part of her team, who was full of helpful ideas and without whose help and advice this text would be so much more cumbersome. I must also thank Jo Clinton Davis, who was the brilliant and sensitive producer of this television series, and her excellent crew, who were so tactful and unobtrusive. Finally, I am grateful to all those at BBC Books, who turned this manuscript around so efficently and quickly.

Introduction

The most important thing that nearly all of us do is to bring a child into this world. There is nothing that changes our lives so completely as having children. Yet some people are denied this enriching experience. Infertile people are not only unable to feel and express the emotions that parenthood brings, they are also barred from contributing to the continuity of human existence. Through our children, fertile people have a kind of immortality which childless couples can often only envy.

This book, which accompanies the television series *Making Babies*, is about the treatment of childlessness by in vitro fertilisation, the 'test tube' baby process. It is not a description of the trials that the admirable men and women filmed in these programmes bravely encountered, because their words express their feelings – and the feelings of thousands of similar infertile couples – far more eloquently than I can. Rather, this book is an attempt to explain my personal response to the wealth of problems, moral, emotional and technical which present themselves to a doctor practising in this field.

In vitro fertilisation, or IVF as it is called throughout this book, is a treatment designed to help women get pregnant when there is a problem of infertility. Originally, it was seen as a useful way of overcoming blocked fallopian tubes by bypassing them when reconstructive surgery had failed or was impossible. Basically, it involves taking eggs directly out of the uterus, fertilising them outside the body by mixing them with prepared sperm, and then placing any embryo which is formed directly back into the uterus where, hopefully, it may grow into a baby. In order to understand the relevance of the various controversial aspects of this work, it is necessary to understand a bit about this process and some of the details of the work that goes on to achieve it.

IVF works best if there is more than one embryo. This is because, under any circumstances, only about one in five human embryos are capable of implanting and becoming a baby. Consequently, IVF doctors try to fertilise as many eggs as possible, and they then choose the embryos which seem to be growing best, for transfer back into the uterus. Therefore, in order to increase the chance of pregnancy, it is normal practice to transfer more than one embryo simultaneously, assuming of course that more than one egg has fertilised. This practice has disadvantages because, occasionally, all the embryos transferred can implant and several babies could be formed. This is why in the early days of IVF, quadruplets and occasionally quintuplets were conceived after treatment. Such results were often regarded as very newsworthy and attracted a great deal of attention in the press. But this was very stressful for the patient who faced a risky pregnancy and delivery, with a high probability of losing one or all of the babies because of their premature birth. Even after delivery, the problems generated by such pregnancies are far from over. Small babies usually need very expensive intensive care in an incubator. Moreover, if they all survive, caring for a number of small babies (even with nursing help at home – which is practically hardly ever available) is nothing short of a nightmare for most couples, even when the babies are desperately wanted.

Because of all these problems, doctors in Britain almost unanimously agreed that it would be in the best interest of patients to limit the number of embryos transferred to three at most. This voluntary agreement, has been reinforced by the Government's regulatory authority, which oversees IVF in Britain. At Hammersmith and the Royal Masonic Hospitals, where the *Making Babies* series was filmed, the number of embryos we transfer is limited to two in nearly all cases. This is because we are concerned even about causing triplets as they increase the risks in the pregnancy, and their nurture is often very complicated. Limiting the number of embryos that are transferred to two or three raises one of the key ethical problems in IVF. What is the status of the surplus embryos which are left over from the process? Can they be destroyed? Can they be given to other infertile women who are unable to generate their own eggs? Is it ethical to do research on them to improve IVF? Is it wise to freeze them? These issues crop up repeatedly in the discussions in this book and during the care of the men and women featured in this documentary series.

The human, unlike most other mammals, usually only produces (or ovulates, to use the correct expression) one egg in each cycle. That is why twins are a relatively uncommon occurrence after natural conception. To make the ovaries produce more than one egg simultaneously to increase the chance of IVF working, fertility drugs are given to the woman. These drugs are basically similar to the naturally produced hormones which stimulate the ovaries during normal ovulation, but are given in large doses by daily injection for maximum effect. Usually it takes about seven to twelve days of this treatment to stimulate the ovary sufficiently, and, in an average IVF cycle, about ten or more eggs may be collected. Taking fertility drugs is not without risk, as occasionally the ovaries can be overstimulated. This can be dangerous, indeed in rare instances it has been lethal. In order to overcome this problem, it is usual to monitor each patient's treatment carefully by making daily measurements of the ovaries on ultrasound. Some units, such as Hammersmith, also measure daily hormone production from the ovaries by taking blood samples.

Collecting the eggs requires a relatively minor operation. In the early days of IVF, it was invariably done with a comparatively deep general anaesthetic. The ovaries were inspected using a telescope (or laparoscope) inserted into the abdomen through a small incision. Eggs were then sucked out of the ovary by inserting a needle into each fluid-filled bag (the follicle) surrounding each egg and applying gentle suction. Nowadays, egg collection is done using a quicker-acting and lighter anaesthetic, usually with the woman in the hospital for just half a day. Sometimes only a little local anaesthetic is used and the woman stays awake throughout the procedure which takes perhaps 25 minutes. This is because, using the modern ultrasound machine to view the ovaries, it is possible to guide a needle into them via the vagina, which is much easier for the woman. The timing of the egg collection is quite critical. Just a day too early, and the developing eggs that are collected may be immature and will not fertilise. A day too late, and the eggs may have already been shed or be degenerate.

Once eggs are obtained, prepared sperm are mixed with each egg in a glass dish. Ordinary seminal fluid will not do for fertilisation. The freshly produced semen has to be carefully filtered and the sperm washed free of any débris, dead sperm, or white blood cells. After this fairly involved preparation, there sometimes may not be enough sperm for fertilisation to occur. Although fertilisation is the result of a single sperm penetrating a single egg, several hundred thousand sperm are usually needed to ensure the maximum chance of fertilisation. Even when there are plenty of sperm and the eggs are entirely healthy, it is very unusual for all the eggs to fertilise. This is why we try to collect as many eggs as possible, so that we can be sure of getting at least one or more embryos.

After fertilisation, embryos are cultured – usually for two or three days – in special media, which are fluids made artificially by laboratory staff to closely resemble the body fluids with which an embryo would normally come into contact. These media contain the nutrients that the embryo needs for growth. Once the embryo is placed into them, it will be stored in a culture oven and kept at body temperature. Here an environment can be provided which mimics conditions normally found inside the human body.

After embryo growth, and whilst the embryos are still completely invisible to the naked eye, they are inspected under a microscope. Assuming that more than one egg has fertilised, the two or three best embryos are selected for transfer and, if things have gone according to plan, the woman is telephoned and recalled to the clinic. The transfer is usually an extremely quick procedure which requires the woman to lie upon a couch for a few minutes. The embryos are loaded into a fine plastic tube and squirted very gently into the uterus through the cervix. This is nearly always completely painless and afterwards she can go home. Although this may be a very simple part of the procedure it is extremely stressful. Even with embryos replaced this way into the uterus, only one-quarter of women will become pregnant. No matter how carefully women are counselled about their embryo transfer, and no matter how vigorously they are warned that there is only about a one in four chance of success, nearly all patients fantasise that they are pregnant after embryo transfer.

Ten to fifteen days after the transfer, blood samples are usually taken to see if there is evidence of a pregnancy. If this test is positive, arrangements are made for an ultrasound scan about two weeks later, so that the presence of a growing baby can be confirmed.

Put like this the procedure sounds blindingly simple but, in practice, IVF is still a highly enigmatic treatment. Women who are least expected to get pregnant sometimes meet with stunning success. Others who we feel are certain to succeed, fail unexpectedly. Unfortunately, IVF is like a monstrous obstacle race and failure can occur at any of the many stages.

For some women, the ovaries may not produce eggs, in spite of heavy stimulation. This distressing occurrence is more common in older women, but it does occur from time to time with younger women whose ovaries are apparently working normally. If no eggs are produced, plans for an egg collection are abandoned, and careful review is needed. We find with other women, after giving the drugs for a short while, that the ovaries are responding too vigorously. This situation, called hyper-stimulation, is potentially hazardous and so the drugs have to be stopped and treatment rescheduled. Occasionally, treatment stops abruptly at a later stage: an attempt at egg collection is made because the ovaries appear to have responded to stimulation, but repeated aspiration reveals no eggs in any of the follicles.

Once eggs are collected, we may find that on the day selected for transfer – and in spite of previous tests being normal – the spermatozoa are of such poor quality that fertilisation is unlikely to occur. Even in completely healthy couples, usually only about 60% of the eggs will fertilise – this is usually as much to do with egg quality (which can vary quite considerably and unexpectedly) as it is to do with sperm. Even if fertilisation rates are good, it is extremely common for only a few, or even none, of the embryos to develop properly, in which case a transfer cannot be done.

But one of the most distressing and common situations is that, having sailed right through all the stages of IVF, including having had apparently perfectly healthy embryos transferred, vaginal bleeding starts about six to ten days later. Alternatively, the menstrual period may be delayed by a few days and most women inevitably find this extraordinarily difficult. Perhaps the worst situation is to get pregnant, rejoice over having a positive pregnancy test and possibly a positive ultrasound scan, and then to miscarry. This depressing event is quite common after IVF and is devastating when it occurs.

Although IVF was originally invented for blocked tubes, it is extraordinarily useful for male problems. This is because fertilisation rates can sometimes be artificially improved by manipulating the sperm in various ways during their culture. IVF is also increasingly used for many problems which cause poor ovulation, because the drugs given during IVF can force the ovary to yield some of its eggs in many of these cases. Infertility is often caused by problems in both partners simultaneously – for example, poor sperm production in the man married to a woman with scarred but not totally blocked fallopian tubes. IVF is particularly useful in such cases, as it is for some couples where the cause of the infertility remains obscure in spite of extensive investigation.

IVF is sometimes thought of as the answer to all infertility problems, but there are many people for whom this treatment is unsuitable. It is generally unhelpful when the ovaries cannot be made to produce eggs – either because there are none left in the ovaries, or because the ovaries are unable to respond to hormonal stimulation. It is true that patients in this situation can be treated using a donated egg from another woman, but sadly egg donation is difficult for the donor and donated eggs are in extremely short supply. There are also many women who have a severely damaged uterus – perhaps because of previous infections and damage to the endometrium, the lining of the womb into which a developing embryo implants. Uterine scarring is common following some operations for benign tumours such as fibroids, and women with a very scarred uterus are unlikely to carry a pregnancy successfully under many circumstances. Some women are born with a congenitally deformed uterus – another cause of infertility which is generally unhelped by IVF. For some of these patients, the only solution to this is for another woman to bear their baby, possibly produced from an egg removed from the patient's ovary. Surrogacy, which is what this way of getting a baby is called, is fraught with risks for the altruistic mother who offers her womb, who may find herself feeling very maternal towards the baby she has to give up.

There are a number of alternatives to IVF. One of these, which has received much publicity, is GIFT. GIFT stands for Gamete IntraFallopian Transfer. With its use, the ovaries are stimulated to produce many eggs just as they are for IVF. Under an anaesthetic, the eggs are collected, mixed immediately with sperm and then placed back into one of the fallopian tubes during the same operation. It is widely used for unexplained infertility and for some cases of male infertility. It is mostly used by those units who are not as successful with IVF as they are with GIFT. It saves having a laboratory in which to culture embryos, but it is not nearly as good a treatment, and is just as demanding and expensive. It is obviously better to transfer embryos knowing that fertilisation and embryo development is normal, rather than unfertilised eggs which may or may not develop further. I shall not be dealing with GIFT in any great detail. If it raises any ethical issue at all, it is simply the question of whether its use is justified when better treatments are available. In my view, most GIFT attempts are something of a waste of resources because IVF gives better information and generally has more chance of producing a baby in good units. I think it a pity that a number of NHS units are using GIFT, and thus offering an expensive second-class treatment, simply because they do not have IVF facilities. This seems to me to be a highly undesirable way of spending what limited public funding is available to help infertile couples. The other alternative to IVF which is worth consideration occasionally is intrauterine insemination, or IUI. IUI is far cheaper than GIFT or IVF and involves placing washed and prepared sperm into the uterine cavity at around the time of ovulation. IUI is most successful when the ovaries are stimulated to produce more than one egg. A limitation is that, as with IVF, care is needed not to overstimulate egg production because there will be a risk of multiple birth.

IVF implies many difficult social and moral dilemmas. It is about these difficult decisions that this book is written. Some of them involve how we decide whether or not infertility is important enough in human terms – a sufficiently serious medical condition – to justify the funding and the resources that are needed for it. Others concern our attitudes to family values, because IVF sometimes requires an egg or sperm donated from another individual. Since IVF is increasingly used for men and women with totally unrelated serious medical conditions, ethical questions are now being raised as to whether it is appropriate to help somebody have a child, when that child is quite likely to be orphaned. Important eugenic issues are also raised. IVF can now help prevent a number of genetic diseases, by selecting healthy embryos free of a specific condition such as muscular dystrophy. Is this a permissible use of technology, and can the screening net be widened to conditions which merely cause mild ill-health? IVF could soon be used to introduce genes to enhance the embryo. What about genetic engineering to improve desirable characteristics, such as intelligence and strength? Most people seem to throw their hands up in horror at the idea, but why should we not try to improve the lot of our children? Sex selection is also possible using IVF, and there are a number of concerns about this which will be examined in this book. Finally, IVF gives doctors access to the human embryo. Research on the human embryo can be done which will greatly improve medical knowledge and thus health. Is this laudable end justified by the means?

Over the last eighteen years, since Louise Brown, the first test-tube baby, was born, there has been a huge amount of ethical debate concerning IVF. All this culminated in 1990, with Britain being the first country to legislate on in vitro fertilisation treatments and on related research on embryos. Parliament felt supportive towards IVF and approved of the research done so far to improve it. In its 1990 Human Fertilisation and Embryology Act, the Government established a regulatory body, the Human Fertilisation and Embryology Authority – or HFEA for short. The HFEA is the body most concerned with the ethical issues raised in this book. It is empowered to inspect and license individual IVF clinics and to ensure that the work with patients and the research conducted in those units is done within the law and to approved ethical standards. It has considerable powers. It keeps records from all the IVF centres and supervises their results. It has the ability to close a clinic which operates consistently below the standards the HFEA sets. It can also initiate criminal proceedings against those practitioners who break the law. One of the questions that I shall be asking in this book is whether the HFEA is really doing an effective job.

Perhaps I may conclude this introduction with a personal note. I helped make this television series with considerable misgivings. In fact, I spent several weeks debating with colleagues and patients before agreeing to allow the BBC crews into the IVF unit. There are considerable ethical problems in filming medical treatments, as any treatment causes great anxiety to the people concerned and the camera is an added intrusion. Going through a treatment like IVF, which involves aspects of our lives which are often the most private and sensitive, is always exceptionally delicate. IVF is also an emotional rollercoaster; one moment the treatment seems to be working, another moment and all is despair. To go through such treatments under a television camera and allow your intimate feelings to be filmed, requires great courage. This book is written with great respect for all people who elect to go through this demanding treatment, but with particular admiration for the generous couples filmed during their treatment. They felt that by making their problem public they would be helping the many other thousands of infertile men and women who seek treatment in Britain. I believe that their participation in these programmes is an important contribution. Their stories are eloquent evidence and they will persuade people who watch of the need to take infertility seriously. Their testimony will, I am sure, help maintain the service and improvements in IVF in this country.

Chapter One

Resources

The human species, Homo sapiens, is one of the most infertile of all mammals. For most couples, regular sexual activity only gives a chance of about 18% each month of a successful pregnancy. Thus it takes an average of at least three to four months for fertile couples to conceive — less fertile people frequently take longer before their efforts are rewarded with conception, and at least 10% of healthy men and women take longer than a year for the pleasure of sex to bear fruit.

The reasons for the unusual subfertility of humans are many. Women, unlike most lower mammals, only produce a single egg, and that at most once a month. Each healthy man, with a single orgasm, ejaculates enough spermatozoa to produce a pregnancy in all the healthy women of child-bearing age in Western Europe. But most of these sperm are either so abnormal in shape or chemical composition, or move so sluggishly that proper fertilisation is impossible. Moreover, once an egg is fertilised and a human embryo is formed, there is only about a 20% chance of pregnancy ensuing. Four-fifths of all human embryos are lost in the first few days after conception, before implantation in the mother's womb. Even when implantation has occurred, the trials of the embryo are not over. Human miscarriage is a common event, and it is likely that between 10–15% of early pregnancies will abort spontaneously for reasons which are still largely obscure.

Just why so many human eggs and sperm are infertile, and why so many of our embryos are so abnormal that they are incapable of further development is still something of a mystery. Certainly, there is no other animal species that I know of where this situation pertains to such a large degree. The mystery is gradually being unravelled by modern biological science, and in later chapters of this book I shall return to some of the causes and how they make an impact on modern fertility treatment and in vitro fertilisation.

In addition to the 'normal' reasons for infertility, humans frequently suffer from disease processes which make infertility very much more likely. Perhaps the commonest problem is a pathological process causing significant reduction in the number of sperm produced by the testicle. Fertile males regularly produce an ejaculate of some 5 millilitres (about a teaspoonful) of fluid containing 180–350 million sperm. In 40% of infertile couples there is a marked reduction in total sperm count, with fewer than 20 million sperm being produced in each millilitre of seminal fluid. Depression of sperm function will also frequently occur if more than average numbers of sperm are not moving properly. Whilst it is possible for a man to impregnate his partner with only a single viable sperm, infertility is a common result when the numbers of sperm are severely reduced. There are many reasons why the production of sperm by a man may be reduced by disease; these include old infections or damage of the testicle, drugs, smoking or other environmental poisons, stress or partial blockage of the fine tubes which lead from the testis to the outside world. However, the most striking feature of most male infertility is that in many men who have decreased sperm production, the cause is usually quite unknown.

In recent years, there has been some publicity in the press given to the fact that men worldwide seem to be much more prone to have 'poor' sperm counts than previously. Perusal of many records from sperm counts from numerous infertility clinics all over Europe suggests that poor sperm production is increasingly common. Records from both Scandinavia and from Britain seem, at first sight, to indicate that human male infertility may be on the increase. The extent of this supposed increasing subfertility of the male population is a source of much dispute, but scientists who believe that male infertility is increasing argue that the reasons for this may be due to changes in our environment. In particular, the widespread use of substances such as insecticides (which are known to depress testicular function) is thought to be having an effect on the overall fertility of us all. Some research workers have argued that male infertility is on the increase because there are numerous chemicals common in our environment which are having a deleterious effect. One group of chemicals which is thought to be particularly important is the oestrogens – essentially female hormones – which are leeching into the water supply because of a number of commercial chemical processes. Such environmental influences ought also to affect animal fertility, particularly domestic and farm animals, but there is fairly limited serious evidence of a reduced fertility in cattle and other animals. It may be, of course, that human production of sperm is a peculiarly sensitive process; a further example of man's natural tendency towards infertility.

Women are prone to many disease processes which cause subfertility. The commonest cause of female infertility worldwide is failure to produce fertile eggs. Ovulatory failure can occur for many reasons. Most of these are due to subtle changes in hormonal control of the ovary. Occasionally, the ovary can just run out of eggs earlier in reproductive life than normal. A very common cause of infertility is damage to fallopian tubes. Such damage frequently follows pelvic infection, in some cases caused by transmission of bacteria during sexual intercourse, in others by a number of different types of bacteria which infect the blood supply temporarily. Pelvic infection is particularly common in some parts of the world such as Africa. Estimates of the incidence of tubal damage in Africa vary, but tubal disease may account for up to 60% of infertility in

African and Caribbean women. Much of this damage is due to sexually transmitted disease, particularly gonorrhoea. (Gonorrhoea is also an important cause of male infertility, for this infection can cause scarring and blockage of the ducts which lead from the testis.) A third cause of female infertility is damage or disease of the uterus. The lining of the uterus, the endometrium, can become scarred as a result of infection during pregnancy, particularly failed pregnancy such as miscarriage. After a pregnancy, retained pieces of placental (afterbirth) tissue can get infected, particularly if medical attempts are made to evacuate the uterus by scraping it out. This is done to curtail bleeding but can cause scarring resulting in adhesions forming inside the uterine cavity. This may prevent any embryo subsequently arriving in the uterine cavity from implanting there. Benign tumours of the uterus, such as fibroids, are also common, particularly in older women. It has been estimated that up to 30–40% of women develop benign fibroids in their uterus as they get older. Such tumours can occupy space in the uterine cavity, resulting in their distorting it and preventing an embryo from developing normally.

Apart from organic disease causing infertility, there are sexual problems which can cause reproductive dysfunction. Human sexual activity is dominated by powerful emotional and psychological factors. As far as we understand, sex is not exactly a cerebral event in most lower animals. It does not appear that animals spend a great deal of time thinking about sex. Preoccupation with sex dominates much of human existence and it is constantly surprising how frequently sexual problems complicate the lives of ordinary people. Sometimes these problems result in infertility; for example, failure to ejaculate successfully in the right place causes infertility in about 3% of couples.

Although the average life-span is now over seventy-five years, the average human female will be capable of

Tania and Ray

Tania, with her partner Ray, had been trying for a baby for some years. Her only child, a boy from her marriage, had been born eleven years earlier and lives with her. Tania is a bubbly and happy individual working as a teacher's assistant in a local primary school. Ray, her partner who was very supportive, works within the fire brigade. The couple had had the sadness of a series of lost pregnancies.

Tania had had a pregnancy in her right tube (a so-called ectopic pregnancy) a few years before I met her. Ectopic pregnancy can be a life-threatening condition, because if the pregnancy bursts the tube, severe internal bleeding can occur so quickly that the results can be fatal. On this occasion, an emergency operation saved Tania's life but the tube had to be removed by the surgeon. After about another year of trying for a baby, Tania conceived again. The news was broken to Tania that this time she had another ectopic pregnancy but in her remaining fallopian tube. An attempt was made to save the tube by injecting the ectopic pregnancy. To do this a telescope was inserted into Tania's abdomen under an anaesthetic and a substance capable of killing the early pregnancy was injected into the pregnancy sac through the wall of the tube, saving Tania from a major operation. An anxious time now followed to see whether the ectopic pregnancy stopped growing, because this kind of injection does not always work. Luckily there were no complications. After two more years of trying, Tania was overjoyed to find that she was able to tell Ray that she was pregnant once more. An ultrasound scan suggested that the baby was growing, but after three months Tania started bleeding and miscarried her baby. In spite of this setback, Tania showed the typical determination shared by so many patients I see. Despite the fear of knowing that she might have to cope with another lost pregnancy, she continued to try to conceive and a few months later Tania missed her period. A pregnancy test was positive, but unbelievably she subsequently found she had another ectopic. Another operation was needed as an emergency. This time her remaining tube was so badly damaged it had to be completely removed and Tania was effectively sterilised.

Some nine months after this, Tania and Ray came to me for the first time. I was impressed by her determination and courage. IVF was the only chance for her and Ray to have children together. Wrongly, I believe, the NHS would not pay for this in spite of all the hardship she had already experienced. She had only modest savings and insisted on private treatment. At that time we had no more charitable funding so were unable to help her financially.

However, the IVF did not go that smoothly. Stimulation with the drugs had to be cancelled because her ovaries overstimulated. Treatment had to be cancelled for safety and was restarted a month later. This time, after further drug treatment, enough eggs were obtained and two embryos were transferred. Fourteen days later we were able to tell Tania that she was pregnant. She was overjoyed to find that both had implanted and she had twins, but started losing a little blood from the vagina at about two months. This was extremely stressful and all too reminiscent of her previous experiences in the earlier pregnancies. She spent a month in hospital before the bleeding finally stopped. The twins were delivered close to term, but even then things were really difficult. The first baby, a girl, was delivered quickly. The second baby, a boy, got stuck during delivery and only after complications could he be released. He was very shocked and was rushed to the neonatal unit. It was only after a week that Tania could be sure that both her babies were well.

having children for only half this time. Women are generally only fertile from about the age of sixteen to forty-five. Estimates of the number of women in Britain between these ages are put at about 11.7 million. As about 10% of couples have problems in conceiving, we can assume that in the UK about 1.1 million women might experience infertility at some time. If we also assume, at a rough guess, that at least half the women of child-bearing age want a family, we might estimate that there are probably close to 600,000 women in this country who are infertile. Here is a cruel paradox. Every infertile couple is led to believe that if all else fails, in vitro fertilisation (IVF) will provide the answer to their prayers. Interest in IVF has been immense. Media interest in IVF and pressure from the medical community in general has led people to believe that it is the answer to this huge health problem. The reality is very different. Only a tiny fraction of those potentially needing this treatment have received it – about 18,000 treatment cycles were done in Britain last year, and in the last five years some 7,000 babies have been born after IVF. Probably around 1% of couples who might benefit have actually had one successful treatment. IVF is truly a very privileged treatment indeed.

To make matters worse, most of those receiving IVF in the last five years received treatment chiefly because they could pay for it. Probably less than 10% of IVF in Britain is done on a National Health Service basis. Neither do private medical insurance companies, such as BUPA, fund IVF treatment. Indeed in Britain it is increasingly difficult to get any of these advanced infertility treatments on a free basis. (Most of the couples we filmed in this television series had to pay for their treatment, except when our own unit was able to provide charitable funds from its hard-pressed budget.)

People may say, why should infertile people get their medical treatment for free? Nobody dies from infertility. For that matter, nobody suffers physical pain through it either. After all, infertility isn't a disease, it is repeatedly said.

Such statements, commonly expressed, show a widespread lack of understanding about what it means to be infertile. Infertility actually causes most of its victims extraordinary pain, a pain moreover which is private and difficult to express (and therefore to resolve) because it is so personal. Most couples when they first realise that they are finding it difficult to conceive just feel anxious. This anxiety soon gives way to feelings of inadequacy and loss of self-esteem. Sometimes the feelings of worthlessness can lead people into believing that their partner would be far better off with another person. Guilt is another strong emotion that many individuals suffer. It is very common for an infertile man or woman to believe that they have brought this state of affairs upon themselves, by some action in the distant past. In practice this is rarely the case, but reassurance by doctors does not always make such feelings diminish. In some cases, childlessness leads to recrimination between partners – perhaps a sense of blame or deprivation, which of course can be deeply corrosive of marital relationships. Various studies have also shown that sexual feelings and sexual performance are affected by being infertile. It is extremely common for women to feel that there is little point in sex any longer. Some feel that they 'are just an empty vessel'. Conversely, men sometimes find that they are unable to sustain an erection and become impotent for a period. Changes in sexual relationships are particularly common during periods of increased awareness of infertility, for example, when going through investigations to ascertain the cause. Another very common negative emotion is a feeling of isolation. For most couples in their mid-thirties, when infertility is most important, social contact means talk of babies, of children, of schools and education. Infertile couples are often deeply threatened by this because they cannot take part in normal social contacts. Infertile women frequently find themselves unable to walk into a room where there are pregnant women. Such feelings may be brought to crisis point when, for example, a younger fertile sister gets pregnant, or parents ask why they are not 'trying for a baby'. Visits to hospital for infertility tests may be particularly difficult, when the infertile patient finds herself in a general clinic where there are women attending for antenatal care, and others arriving to discuss termination of an unwanted pregnancy. Not surprisingly, all these unhappy emotions very frequently lead to frustration and are expressed in anger. Anger may be inwardly directed, but equally may be directed at a clinic which is seen to be less efficient, or a doctor who is perceived to be apparently uncaring or 'incompetent'.

Recognition of the social and emotional consequences of infertility is not new. They are as old as the Bible itself. In the Old Testament, no fewer than three out of the four matriarchs – Sarah, Rebecca, Leah and Rachel – are affected by infertility. Biblical accounts show remarkable insights into the consequences and the effect on family. In Sarah's case, her husband Abraham has been repeatedly promised by God that his seed will become as multitudinous as the 'stars in the firmament'. God also promises him wealth and substance, at one point consoling him 'Fear not Abram, I am thy shield, thy reward shall be exceeding great'. To this, Abraham piteously replies, 'O Lord, what wilt thou give me, seeing that I go childless...?' Later in Genesis, Sarah says to Abraham, 'Behold now, the Lord hath restrained me from childbearing; go in, I pray thee, unto my handmaid; perhaps I shall be builded up through her.' The Biblical passage is remarkable because it shows that Sarah is prepared to go to extraordinary lengths for her husband to have children. She is effectively commissioning a surrogacy arrangement with her own servant, Hagar, an arrangement which, incidentally, brings terrible grief after Ishmael is born. Both he and Hagar are rejected and sent out to die in the desert. The passage is also evocative because of the phrase that Sarah uses: 'perhaps I may be builded up through her'. Sarah's self-esteem is at rock-bottom and she considers that she would have more status if a child is born, by whatever means.

The second matriarch to be affected by infertility is Rebecca, Sarah's daughter-in-law. Only after a long time trying does Rebecca fall pregnant, when she has the twins Esau and Jacob, who incidentally spend a lifetime fighting each other.

When Jacob marries first Leah and later Rachel, the question of infertility is brought to a head. Leah is ugly and unfavoured but she is highly fertile, giving birth to four sons in quick succession. In the meantime Rachel, who is beautiful and clearly Jacob's favourite, remains sterile. The Bible tells us that Rachel 'envied her sister' and cries to Jacob with a cry which echoes down the ages, 'Give me children, or else I die'. Rachel can find no point in continued existence, whatever her favoured status. Jacob's reaction to Rachel's outburst is telling: 'Am I in God's stead, who has withheld from thee the fruit of the womb?' Jacob is reacting angrily and appears to lay the blame for Rachel's unhappiness at her door. Could there be a more poignant and succinct account of the isolation and anger that results from childlessness?

One might believe that things have improved greatly in 5,000 years since Biblical times. That in our society, in the West, childlessness no longer has the stigma which Rachel or Sarah felt. Sadly this is far from the case. In many, if not in most countries of the world, infertility is worse than mere hardship. In many Muslim countries a man may divorce an infertile wife if she is without child, irrespective of whether the cause of the infertility is thought to be a female or a male problem. Some years ago I came across a princess married to a ruler in one of the Gulf States. She lived in some splendour in the Royal Palace and had had two daughters by her husband, the Ruler. In spite of eight further years trying, she never conceived the wanted son and heir, indeed never conceived at all. She submitted to all sorts of investigations and the indignities that sometimes can follow such tests. Nothing wrong was found with her. Eventually, with extreme difficulty and after much negotiation, we were able to persuade the Sheikh to give a sperm sample. This showed severe male infertility and probable damage from an old gonorrhoea infection. In spite of intense and delicate explanation from us, we were quite unable to persuade the Sheikh that the problem lay with him. Eventually, this wife was expelled from the Palace, abandoning not merely her privileged life but also her two much-loved daughters aged ten and eight. Remarriage brought for the Ruler no further children, but still we were not allowed to offer him treatment. In most parts of Africa, very similar attitudes still prevail. In much of Nigeria, after all a relatively developed and industrialised country, female infertility is virtually a death sentence. Many couples there test their fertility by trying to conceive before marriage; marriage will follow only after fecundity is demonstrated. As marriage may be the only chance for a woman to live with some economic security – for example, with a roof over her head – a barren woman can effectively be an outcast thrown onto the charity of society. In many parts of Asia, for example, rural India or Bangladesh, children are the only insurance people have for maintenance in their old age. Where incomes are not much above subsistence level and with no formal state support for old people, a large family will be the only riches in some agricultural communities. Small wonder then that infertility is such a serious problem to sufferers, and why incidentally, over-population is so impossible to control.

Perhaps the biggest hurdle that couples face in the United Kingdom is this idea that infertility is not a 'disease'. Two important consequences follow the failure to recognise that infertility is not caused by a disease process. Firstly, it means that health care resources need not be provided in so many cases. Secondly it results in infertility being treated without a diagnosis being made. Invariably, infertility means that something is wrong, yet far too often the cause is left undiagnosed. Consequently, treatment is haphazard and conducted on an irrational basis. The ultimate irrationality is the inappropriate offer of IVF. A woman can walk into most IVF clinics and ask for, and obtain (if she can afford it), IVF. This is akin to the patient with pain in the chest walking into her GP's surgery and asking for radiotherapy. But pain in the chest may be due to a chest infection, in which case antibiotics would be called for. Chest pain may be due to indigestion, in which case an antacid may be needed. Alternatively it may be due to problems with the heart, in which case coronary artery surgery may be needed. The chance that it is due to lung cancer is remote and therefore a demand for immediate radiotherapy would seem laughable to any serious or responsible doctor. Yet the infertile patient is frequently denied logical or methodical assessment. She can walk in and demand IVF not least because the medical services of the State have washed their hands of her condition.

This may seem extraordinary, but this genuinely happens far too frequently, occasionally even in the public sector. There is at least one large NHS infertility clinic in London, attached to a major teaching hospital, where the standard policy now is to offer IVF simply because this is seen to be a virtual panacea for nearly all cases of infertility. No detailed investigations are offered, with the excuse that they cost money. Laparoscopy (inspection of the uterus, tubes and ovaries – the standard infertility test) is not done; neither, for example, is a womb X-ray to see if the uterus is undamaged. If in this particular unit, after IVF has failed in spite of transferring an embryo to the uterus, the uterus is found to be abnormal, this is regarded as simply bad luck. Matters are often no better in the private sector. Most private IVF clinics are free-standing; that is to say they are IVF units pure and simple, often not set up to conduct comprehensive infertility care. In such places, IVF is bound to be offered routinely because it is much simpler for the clinic to conduct such treatments. Patients are increasingly at risk of exploitation because commercial convenience may lead private clinics to offer their standard therapy.

Leaving aside potentially unnecessary treatment and the issue of the amount of likely distress that may be caused, all this, of course, is wasteful of resources. A cycle of IVF can cost anything from £1400–2200, but this figure does not include the cost of drugs needed to make the ovaries sufficiently hard to produce several eggs at once. Although natural cycle IVF (IVF without any extra drugs, leaving the patient to produce one egg for collection naturally) can be done, it has very low success rates. The drugs used to stimulate the ovaries are made up in glass ampoules. Each ampoule costs about £10 and usually an average of thirty are needed. Many patients need sixty or seventy ampoules in all, at a basic cost of around £700. To make matters worse, most patients in Britain are asked to get their drugs supplied on prescription from their general practitioner. In the case of NHS patients, this saves hospital pharmacies from prescribing from their hard pressed drug budget (all hospitals try to keep pharmacy costs as low as possible). In the case of private clinics, this reduces the overall cost to the patient, who can frequently get her drugs from her GP who is likely to be sympathetic to her plight. However, this greatly adds to the drug bill, eventually met by the taxpayer. This is because hospitals get drugs direct from the manufacturer at the basic price, often with a discount. Discounts of this sort can promote a drug company's sales, because their drug representatives will be well aware that hospital prescriptions encourage further sales of their product outside the hospital. GP prescriptions are sold by retail pharmacists in the high street and there is usually a considerable mark-up. An ampoule costing £10 in the hospital pharmacy, may cost twice or even more when dispensed over the counter of the local chemist's shop. Consequently thirty ampoules which might cost £300 if given by a general hospital are likely to cost at least £600 to the NHS. If more of the drug is needed, the costs are consequently even more. Such extra costs might just be acceptable if IVF is really the treatment most likely to be effective. If IVF is offered simply because it is the treatment most readily available, the NHS is left severely out of pocket. It is likely that at least an extra £5 million is spent in the UK in this way annually – enough to give another 5,000 patients one chance at IVF on an NHS basis in NHS hospitals where most offer this treatment on a contract basis.

The cost of IVF is one of the concerns that many ordinary people have when considering it. Most couples realise that, statistically speaking, an IVF treatment cycle is unlikely to work first time; certainly, all responsible clinics are at pains to point this out very carefully. In practice, for the average couple in an average clinic, a single treatment with IVF has odds of 7–1 against producing a baby (roughly 14% chance). Consequently, in such an average clinic, most couples will need to try at least four cycles of IVF just to get a better than evens chance of success. People who would never dream of betting on the Grand National or at a roulette wheel find themselves faced with a divine throw of the biological dice. But rather like the person coming off the street to face the Banker in the casino, the odds are always slightly higher than they seem. In the case of Tania and Ray, (who eventually conceived twins successfully), the cost of IVF was one of the major worries they had. In their first cycle of treatment, the stimulation before IVF failed and treatment had to be cancelled before Tania even managed to go to have her eggs collected. Even though a cancelled cycle like this is never charged at full cost, it does mean extra unexpected and therefore unbudgeted expenses of several hundred pounds.

Very often, the costs involved with IVF persuade a couple to gamble further. A very good example of this is seen with embryo freezing. Most clinics now suggest to couples that any spare embryos produced as a byproduct of IVF are frozen. As we have seen, many eggs are usually collected at IVF, about nine or ten in an average cycle. Typically, 60% of the eggs will fertilise normally after exposure to sperm. As it is unsafe to transfer more than two or three embryos to the uterus simultaneously (for fear of producing triplets or quadruplets), 'spare' embryos are left over after most IVF attempts. A couple has the option of destroying these, donating them for research, or storing them after freezing them.

Frozen embryos can be kept virtually indefinitely in liquid nitrogen, at extremely low temperatures. Mice embryos have now been kept for twenty-five years with not much deterioration after thawing. There is no reason to suppose that human embryos would be any different. In view of all this, it seems sensible to increase the odds of our bet, by freezing any spare embryos for transfer later. This saves the cost of the drugs and most of a treatment cycle, and simply incurs the cost of freezing and a transfer cycle (in most clinics about £500–850) or about half to one-third of a full treatment.

However, freezing does carry significant implications. Apart from the emotional risks in having stored embryos (consider the potential difficulties, for example, if one parent partner dies or there is an acrimonious divorce), there is still a question in my mind as to whether freezing is really safe. What is the evidence that freezing harms human embryos?

There is the recognised fact that embryos are less likely to produce a pregnancy after freezing and thawing. Different clinics produce varying data; because there is no standard way of reporting the results after freezing, it is quite difficult to get an accurate idea of the attrition rate involved in embryo freezing. Collated world figures suggest that less than 3% of embryos after thawing and transfer are likely to produce a baby. By comparison, 'fresh' embryos have at least a 16% chance of being delivered as a baby in any good clinic. This is clear evidence of damage. It is worth looking in detail at the results from one very famous and extremely capable centre in Belgium. These results are from Professor van Steirteghem's team and were published in 1994. He reported clinical results following the freezing of embryos after routine IVF and after treatments for male infertility. I have extracted just the relevant results following freezing after routine IVF in the following table:

Number of embryos frozen	2495	
Number of embryos thawed	969	
Number embryos transferred	253	(26% of embryos thawed)
Number of implanted embryos	29	(11.5% of embryos transferred)
Number of live births	18	(1.8% of embryos thawed)

This is the evidence from a top-class programme. Only 1.8% of frozen/thawed embryos resulted in a baby. Of the thawed embryos, only 26% were even considered potentially viable after thawing. Only 11.5% of thawed embryos implanted (about half what would be expected at Hammersmith Hospital with fresh embryos – we have around 22% implantation rate per embryo). It is impossible not to draw the conclusion that freezing damages a substantial number of human embryos.

Moreover, it is damage which can clearly be seen down a microscope. At the stage when most embryo freezing is done, the embryo is a clump of around four to eight cells. Microscopic inspection after the thawing of, for example, what was an eight-cell embryo before freezing will show that some of its cells are dying, missing or fragmented. Of course, it is clearly established that an embryo is still perfectly capable of growing into a normal baby after such damage. Indeed, there is incontrovertible evidence that embryo freezing does not increase the risk of there being any abnormality at birth. Several thousand babies have now been delivered after 'life in the deep freeze' and there is no evidence at all of any increase in fetal abnormality. Nonetheless, there is the vague concern that there may be problems in the longer term after freezing as these children grow up.

During the process of embryo freezing, any water in the embryonic cells needs to be first removed. Water left in the cells will form ice crystals. Anyone who has placed a can of fizzy cola in the deepfreeze will know too well that ice expands on thawing and causes the can to burst because of the huge pressure it exerts. Ice crystal formation and subsequent thawing in an embryonic cell can lead to the cell's rupture, or possibly cause damage to the delicate structures inside the cell. In order to overcome the problem of ice formation, embryos are first bathed in a solution of 'antifreeze' to get rid of most of the cellular water. Several such compounds are commonly used in embryo freezing, and perhaps one of the commonest in use is dimethylsulphoxide (or DMSO, as it is commonly called). DMSO is a powerful solvent and can penetrate cell walls very quickly – it is this property which makes for its use as a carrier to deliver other drugs across the skin in some situations. DMSO is also a potential mutagen. In high doses, it has been associated with mutation of the DNA in cells. Moreover, because it is a powerful solvent, it may dissolve other mutagens within it which go on to cause mutation. Such effects might go unnoticed in embryos for a considerable length of time after birth.

Some experienced embryologists have actually recorded visible damage to the cell nucleus after freezing and thawing. The nucleus is the filing cabinet or bookcase of the cell; it is where key messages and directions about the cell's function are composed and transmitted. It is where the DNA is kept. The DNA is the blueprint of the organism, the genetic code which formulates all our inherited characteristics, including which diseases we are likely to be prone to. The damage to the cell nucleus which has been observed has shown that part of the DNA has been excluded from the nucleus and is lying outside the nuclear membrane. This is potentially serious because if the DNA is damaged in this way it would be unlikely to be able to give its complete message normally; part of the blueprint would be missing or damaged. All this, too, could give rise to children who were in some way genetically altered.

The evidence from freezing animal embryos is also worrying. Some recent work by French scientists examined the long-term effect of freezing embryos in mice. They compared adult mice which had been frozen when being cultured at the embryo stage, with mice which had been similarly treated in every way during embryo growth except that they had not been frozen. They reported three possible unexpected differences in the mice which had been frozen during embryo growth. Firstly, they tended to grow fatter than usual in old age. Secondly, some of the frozen mice showed changes in their jaw structure as they grew. Lastly, psychological testing on their behaviour showed that many of the mice which had been frozen exhibited different behavioural patterns. The authors put all this down to a possible genetic effect of freezing. Some scientists, mostly those who freeze human embryos and therefore may not be truly objective, have attempted to debunk this work, despite it being published in one of the world's most authoritative scientific journals, *Proceedings of the National Academy of Sciences*. This is a journal whose editors would be absolutely scrupulous in checking any research they published, because their imprimatur carries considerable weight.

One of the problems with freezing is that if it did cause mutation occasionally, it would be quite unlikely to show these effects in infancy. Mutagenic effects often occur much later in life and are typically shown by a tendency to develop cancers or to be infertile. There are precedents for this. Ionising radiation (such as X-rays) can cause mutation if pregnant animals are exposed during early gestation. The trouble is it can take a very long time for these effects to surface and be documented. It was fifty years before we realised that X-rays during pregnancy increase the chance of exposed offspring developing leukaemia later in life.

I am not saying that embryo freezing causes cancer, infertility or leukaemia. I am simply saying that, to my mind, it is still an experimental procedure and we should be cautious about its use. Certainly I believe that embryo freezing should only be offered to patients when there are no good alternatives. But desperate women, who see a chance of potentially cutting the costs of their treatment, are all too ready to take an extra gamble which they might be more reluctant to take in other circumstances. I also find it unacceptable that many of my colleagues never warn patients that there are some concerns about embryo freezing; in fact there is almost a conspiracy of silence. When I raise objections, I am frequently put down by my colleagues, presumably because I threaten the status quo or undermine a useful commercial enterprise. Indeed, one director of a major private clinic with a large freezing programme recently suggested I was trying to seek attention by 'scaremongering'.

As it happens, there is an extraordinary paradox about this as there is about so much of infertility treatment. Embryo freezing is almost certainly not cost effective. If two or three embryos are frozen and offered later for transfer, the combined chance of their producing a successful pregnancy is no more than 6–9%. At a cost of £600–850 for freezing and transfer, in the more successful clinics it would probably be cheaper to have fresh embryos transferred in a new cycle.

We often hear, of course, that in an ideal world it would certainly be a very good idea to fund IVF on an NHS basis. However, people go on to say, we do not live in an ideal world and there is only a finite amount of money available in the Health Service. The problem is, it is said, that whilst people are dying of kidney failure and we need to make increasing provision for our aging population, it is not justified to spend more money on trivial medical conditions such as infertility. Now, I am not advocating a great expansion of public expenditure on health care, although it is true that we spend less per capita on health in Britain than most European countries. What I do argue is that we could spend what we are spending much more prudently. In its latest reforms of the Health Service, the Government set up an internal market. These have not been wholly in the interest of prudent financial management. Under these reforms, local health authorities are required to provide health care for residents in the area of the country for which they are responsible. They are given a budget and committees within the health authorities (the purchasers) decide if they are going to buy particular services, and from which providers. Some purchasers refuse to 'buy' IVF at all; others have a more liberal attitude. So, whether you are able to get NHS infertility treatment at all depends mostly on your address – hardly a fair way of dividing the taxpayer's investment in health care. The 'providers' are the general hospitals who can tender to provide a particular service, be it IVF or general surgery, under contract for a given number of patients from that health authority. Organisations other than the general hospitals can also tender contracts. In the case of IVF, many of the larger private clinics are competing for contracts within the health service. Sometimes the private clinics have offered their services under contract at quite a high price, certainly higher than many NHS or university hospital providers, perhaps because of a favourable geographical location close to the purchasing authority, or because purchasers (who generally have a poor understanding of the intricacies of IVF and the interpretation of the results that a given clinic may be advertising) are bemused by the apparently favourable information that the private clinics are putting out. In general, most private clinics spend considerable sums of money on promotional material which looks extremely enticing except perhaps to the most discerning reader.

The 'purchaser/provider split' has several unfortunate consequences. Apart from the haphazard, and therefore inherently unfair, level of provision of services, it has resulted in a considerable wastage of money. Purchasers buying IVF from a private clinic may well be paying more than they might from a good district hospital, and the funds that the private clinic receives are basically turned back into profits for the clinics owners and any shareholders. The net result is a drop in investment in the public sector. This is wrong for several reasons.

Firstly, most of the good scientific progress and contributions have always traditionally been made in the public sector in this country, and still are. In the IVF field a survey of published research shows that the public sector has been much more scientifically prolific, which suggests that most useful innovation in the field comes from these centres. Although there are far more private clinics than NHS ones, it is interesting that of the thirty-nine licences for basic research granted by the HFEA, only three are registered in private clinics. To avoid sending patients to public sector units will mean their eventual attrition and lack of further progress in the field in Britain.

The second issue is that by allowing the 'market forces' (so dear to Margaret Thatcher's heart) to operate, IVF actually becomes more costly. It might be thought that the spirit of healthy competition would drive prices down. There is little evidence of this happening in the health care 'market'. What has actually happened in the IVF field is that more and more small units have opened up in competition with each other. General hospitals with minimal expertise, casting around for new areas to market, latch on to IVF, which is sometimes seen as an area in which they might make a killing, because it is apparently highly profitable in the private sector. The competition developing around the area of Hammersmith Hospital, is a case in point. London already has at least twenty-one IVF units – more than enough to cope with any demand. Hammersmith is the biggest in London – indeed, one of the busiest units in the world. It is also one of the more successful. It has a staff of seventy, with the equivalent of four specialist consultants and can provide the whole range of comprehensive infertility treatment. Analysis by the Government's own regulatory body, the Human Fertilisation and Embryology Authority (HFEA), shows that large units are considerably more likely to be successful than small units. This is because there is greater concentration of expertise, better staffing levels, more experience and better laboratories in large units. Just recently, within a few miles of Hammersmith, a new IVF unit has been opened in an NHS hospital. The hospital has no specialist infertility clinic of any renown and, as far as I am aware, has published nothing of scientific merit in recent years in the field. It has no specialist infertility consultants, and certainly could not provide truly comprehensive infertility care. Recently, the hospital concerned was interviewing candidates for the post of embryologist in their new IVF unit. It was reported back to me that one candidate, rather boldly, asked how the new unit intended to compete 'seeing as the Hammersmith Hospital, with its world-class facilities, is on your doorstep'. The reply was, 'we intend to undercut their prices'. Now, as it happens, I do not believe that Hammersmith's prices could be undercut – because it amasses considerable charitable funding and because at Hammersmith all private income is channelled back into the NHS system. It is actually one of the cheapest units in the country, let alone London,which tends to be more expensive than average.

What will be the likely result? Firstly, there will be another IVF unit in London – which frankly is unnecessary. Secondly, within a year or two, this unit is likely to become unprofitable and close – but not before considerable NHS resources have been spent on commissioning it and maintaining its staff, and not before far more patients than necessary are likely to have failed a treatment which would have been better administered in the larger unit.

The paradox is that the internal market, which tends to fragment some health care in this way, actually results in worse treatment, or treatments of all sorts with less expertise. In the field of infertility I believe we could provide a far better organised and efficient service, to more patients, without any extra spending at all. Currently the NHS is wasting money. If any reforms in the provision of care are to be undertaken, the most vital should be the centralisation of resources for such treatments as IVF. Regional services in major centres would be a much better investment for the taxpayer. Considerable expertise could be concentrated there, and the bigger throughput would ensure much more efficient and cheaper medical care. Given proper thought, patients could still experience individualised IVF, and the rationalisation of space, materials and staffing would ensure the best value for money. It would also ensure the best chance of a pregnancy, which is clearly what the patient wants. Certainly it is true that the couple may need to travel a little further for their treatment, but at the end of the journey they know they would be guaranteed the best IVF available – rather than experience the current uncertainties which so many infertile patients face.

One of the biggest difficulties which remains is this. If we do believe that the NHS should be available for IVF treatment, which couples should benefit? We have already seen at the beginning of this chapter that there are possibly 600,000 infertile couples in Britain. Luckily, most of them do not want IVF. If they did, offering each one of them one IVF treatment cycle at current NHS contract rates would cost about £400 million – considerably more if treatment was in private clinics – and at least 1% or more of the total cost of all health care in Britain. Clearly there needs to be rationing somewhere.

Firstly, there should be some proper assessment of the medical condition, that IVF is really the treatment of choice and is genuinely necessary. This is not done in any systematic way at present. Different referring GPs form their own judgment as to whether it is clinically justifiable to send a patient for an IVF attempt. Very often, it is the patient herself (who may certainly not be the best judge of what is the best form of treatment) who pushes for IVF rather than a more suitable, and possibly cheaper, alternative. There should certainly be guidelines for when NHS IVF treatment is to be considered. These could possibly be nationally accepted and be flexible enough to allow for odd circumstances.

One of the problems is that there is a whole range of social issues which complicate the availability and suitability of IVF treatment. For example, should IVF be available to couples who are living together but not formally married? Most people would seem to think this entirely acceptable, but by no means everybody. If a couple is living together, should there be a minimum time-limit on how long they should cohabit in order to ensure that they are genuinely in a stable relationship? At first glance this may seem rational and fair, but it is worth considering that the fertile members of the population do not have to go through any such assessment when they are considering having a baby.

One of the biggest issues is whether a couple should be offered IVF when they have already had a child in that relationship. Most purchasing health authorities are extremely reluctant to consider arranging NHS IVF under such circumstances. This was the concern in Tania's case. In spite of losing four pregnancies and requiring two major operations to save her life, in spite of the continued distress to her and the corrosion of her life, she was not eligible. She had already had a child with her ex-husband and was therefore, according to some arbitrary decisions, not infertile. Too many health authorities – including the one in her area – would not consider her worthy for IVF funding. At first, this may seem a rational decision given her eleven-year-old child. However, it may be that single-child families are significantly dis-advantaged. Many parents feel that their only child is much more lonely and has far more difficulty with developing social relationships. Many couples feel under huge pressure when their only child asks them about a baby brother or sister, and this causes them huge problems. Many couples have told me that being infertile in such circumstances is actually much worse than if they had never had a child at all. One woman said to me (and I have heard this kind of statement in various ways) '...if only I had never had a child; that might have been preferable – at least I would not have known what it was like to have a baby'. Such statements may seem selfish, but there is no doubt about the deep sense of injury and the grief that that couple felt.

If the situation is complicated in couples, these difficulties are pallid compared with the difficulties that single women face. It is a ruling of the regulatory authority, the HFEA, that the welfare of any child born as a result of IVF should be considered when clinicians embark on IVF treatments. From time to time we are asked to provide treatment for single women – for example, with stored frozen sperm after a husband's death – or treatment for a lesbian couple. At first, it would seem that this is a perfect example of where a child is likely to be disadvantaged. No father figure exists and no male sex role model. It is widely believed that children brought up by a lesbian couple may exhibit some profound sexual disturbance. As it happens, there is no serious evidence that children born from single women or to lesbian couples are in any way disadvantaged. Most of the studies which have been done on single-parent families are studies under various conditions of deprivation. There have been no definitive long-term studies of cases where single women could clearly afford to maintain a much-wanted child, or where a lesbian couple were happily providing the parenting required.

At the other end of the scale is the couple who is rather more unlikely than average to get a successful treatment cycle. Thus purchasing authorities are very reluctant to offer IVF treatment to women over forty because they see this as a treatment much more likely to be wasted i.e. not producing a child. Sometimes the decision is even more questionable. In 1995, the health authority in Sheffield decided that it would not offer NHS funding for an IVF treatment for a woman, Mrs F., aged thirty-seven. Their decision appeared to be taken mostly on the grounds that, given her age, treatment was less likely than average to succeed and therefore the money would not be well spent. The woman in question appealed to the courts, but her application to get funding was refused and the decision of the health authority ratified. It is worth taking a look at this decision. In our unit, a woman of thirty-seven would have a 23% chance of having a baby with one IVF cycle; a woman of thirty-six, a 25.5% chance. The difference of less than 2% was, effectively, the difference between funding or not funding. This may be justified, but it is arbitrary. Suppose, instead of being thirty-seven years old, Mrs F. had been thirty-five years old and two stone overweight. Our figure clearly show that her chances of getting pregnant would have been about 14% – almost half the normal chance and substantially less than a woman of thirty-seven. Yet she would have been regarded as completely acceptable for NHS treatment in Sheffield, if not in nearly every health authority in Britain that is prepared to offer this treatment.

Whatever the decision about all these issues, and who is suitable for IVF treatment, previously certain ethical principles were always clear. I was taught firmly as a medical student that NHS treatment was justified if it were justified privately. It was always a firm principle that ability to pay was ethically not a dividing line between those who were suitable for a treatment and those who were not. I was also brought up on the notion that to ignore this principle led to corruption of medical values, that some patients might get a treatment that really wasn't justified simply because they could pay for it. My clinical teachers pointed out firmly to all of us that this was the first line of potential medical exploitation of patients. It seems that perhaps the internal market has changed all that, and that this ethical principle no longer holds good.

No modern society can be completely fair. However, in an ideally fair society, the question of the ability to pay for medical treatment would be a poor criterion in making the decision as to who gets treated. Let us assume that Health Service economics do not exist. Who does merit treatment?

Certain general ethical principles exist. Firstly, there should be respect for the autonomy of the people seeking treatment. I am often faced with particularly desperate couples for whom the only chance of a baby is IVF, but for whom the chance even with this treatment is very poor. I know that in their case IVF is unlikely to succeed because of the medical circumstances. I may also feel, perhaps knowing the couple who are seeking private treatment, that IVF could be too great a financial or psychological burden for them. Nevertheless, ultimately it would be wrong for me to refuse this couple treatment once they are in the position of knowing all the facts which surround their circumstances. They surely have the right to choose. If their autonomy is to be properly respected, the couple must be given all the information possible and then left free to decide for themselves whether or not they have treatment. This is the principle of informed consent. It would certainly be undesirable for the doctor, or for that matter a social worker or a nurse, to decide on a paternalistic basis whether or not a particular infertile couple merits the treatment. Neither the doctor, nurse, social worker nor anyone else can put themselves in the shoes of this couple and say that the distress they feel does or does not justify the gamble they are taking. In this respect, infertility medicine is different from much other medical practice. In other branches of medicine, there may be circumstances where the doctor may need to take decisions to some extent on behalf of the patient. For example, when treating a cancer from which the patient may die, the doctor would be incorrect in not leading a patient towards what he sees as the most suitable decision regarding treatment. In reproductive medicine, though, the decisions are based much more on what qualities of life the couple feel are important to them as people, rather than questions of life or death.

There are two major exceptions to all this. Firstly, a principle of medical treatment should be that, wherever possible, it 'does no harm' and potentially it 'may do good'. Doctors choosing which patients to treat by IVF must first consider the adverse consequences. For example, it seems to me that I would be absolutely right to refuse treatment to a couple if I thought that the risks to their health very greatly outstripped the possible benefits. If I feel deeply uncomfortable about treating a particular couple, then my own autonomy is also deserving of respect. Ultimately I am entitled to refuse a treatment if I think it is wrong to do it. Let me give two examples. The first concerns a woman for whom, for various reasons, there would be a serious risk to her life if she underwent treatment. I recently saw a woman who had previously had a major venous thrombosis (clots in her veins) and subsequently a stroke that almost caused her death. To give such a person the drugs needed to drive the ovaries to produce eggs could have fatal effects. Nevertheless, she was desperate for a child and requested IVF, knowing, as a highly informed and intelligent woman, all the risks she might be taking. I felt obliged to refuse her treatment because I did not feel I could take the responsibility for the huge risk she would be running, even though she verbally absolved me from any suggestion that an accident would be any other than her own fault. Another example where I am even more sure that one is justified in withholding treatment is in the situation where I, as the doctor, have strong suspicions that any child born might be seriously at risk, for example, from child abuse. The HFEA has as its guideline that physicians treating infertile couples with IVF should always bear in mind the welfare of any child born as a result of the treatment. To my mind, this is a rule which is practically very limited because most of the time it will never be possible to forecast the long-term outcome in anyone's circumstances. However, when a child is likely to be in physical danger, it would certainly seem sensible to refuse treatment.

An example of the question of the right to decide treatment came up recently. It resulted in decisions which, at the time, caused me considerable distress. It concerned the question of whether or not we should treat a woman, who I shall call Sheila, who was HIV positive and therefore at risk of developing AIDS at a later date.

Sheila had, when she was nineteen, been a drug user. At that time she was heavily under the influence of a boyfriend who almost certainly infected her with the Human Immune-deficiency Virus. Some years later, she escaped from her boyfriend's clutches and kicked the heroin use. When we first met, she had been free of any drugs for eight years, and HIV positive for ten. For the last five years she had been in a totally supportive relationship. Because they knew that she was HIV positive, the couple had been using safe sex since they had met. Her partner was free of the virus. Although unmarried, this relationship was clearly very stable, and the two of them came to consult me about their infertility. Both desperately wanted children, and it was completely clear that her partner, whom I shall call Alan, very much wanted her child. Sheila had blocked tubes, and had been promised infertility treatment at another well-known teaching hospital in London when she visited it as an outpatient. When an X-ray showed that her tubes were blocked, however, they refused to do a laparoscopy but gave no concrete grounds for their refusal. Such behaviour is, in my experience, not uncommon in this speciality of medicine because, even amongst doctors, infertility is sometimes not seen as being sufficiently important to take seriously. At the clinic in this hospital, they advised her to go for IVF, but then pointed out that this was not a treatment they did themselves. Moreover, they were relatively unprepared to suggest where she might go for treatment. Neither did they warn her that, because she was HIV positive, she might find it difficult to get this treatment.

Sheila made an appointment to see me privately. At first I felt clear in my own mind that I was relatively sure that I would not want to offer her IVF, and told her this. Nevertheless, I thought it would certainly be right to see what was causing her infertility, and to see if it was correctable. After all, had she had normal fallopian tubes, the choice would have been hers alone whether or not she could try for a pregnancy. I agreed to her request for a private laparoscopy, so that the NHS would not be paying for her investigations, but did not charge her any medical fees. Laparoscopy revealed that any attempt at tubal surgery would be pointless – there was not the slightest chance of it restoring her fertility because her tubes were hopelessly damaged. Her only chance of a baby would be by IVF.

The three of us, Sheila, Alan and I, retraced the arguments for and against IVF. Discussion was easy and without embarrassment because they were so open. Against treatment was the idea that Sheila was even-tually likely to contract AIDS and die of this disease. Her child could be motherless within a year or two of birth. Then there was a finite possibility that the baby could be born with this infection, and could also die within a few years of birth. It was difficult to get an accurate estimate of the risk of the baby being born infected, but there might have been a 10–15% risk. To some extent this risk could be kept in check by not allowing the baby to be born vaginally and doing a Caesarean section instead. With this and by giving antiviral drugs during pregnancy the risk of transferring the virus might be kept to around 7%, but nobody I had carefully consulted beforehand could give a clear indication of the precise risk. In favour of treatment was the knowledge that many people have children knowing there may be reasons why they may die in the near future. Many others quite responsibly have children knowing that, because they carry a gene for a fatal inherited disease, the baby may have up to a 50% chance of dying within a year or so of birth. This is a gamble they take – as I believe they are entitled to take – in the hope of having normal offspring. There was also the knowledge that there is increasing evidence that some people who are HIV positive remain so for very extended periods of time, without necessarily developing full-blown AIDS. Sheila had been completely well for ten years with a normal blood count, and might remain well for very much longer. But above all, there was my increasing impression after four lengthy out-patient sessions that Sheila and Alan were highly responsible and caring people, who loved each other, who had thought it all through and wanted the chance of a baby. It was clear that had Sheila been normally fertile, she and her partner would not be sitting in front of me, requesting my permission for IVF, for which they wanted to pay. I was sure that I should respect their autonomy. First, I said, I needed to contact the regulatory authority, the HFEA and also the Chairman of own local Ethics Committee. Then I would present their case to our IVF team at one of our formal monthly meetings, when situations of this sort are discussed.

The representative of the HFEA said that this, in principle, was the kind of decision they had discussed in their committees. They were worried about the problems involved but ultimately felt that this was a decision which had to be taken by the doctor together with the patients. The HFEA therefore raised no objection. The Chairman of our Ethics Committee was in favour of treatment, as indeed were several senior colleagues with whom I raised the issue.

The following Monday I went to our team meeting feeling confident and buoyed up in the knowledge that I was undoubtedly doing the right thing by offering Sheila the treatment. I had little anticipated the storm that erupted. I have always felt that when there were difficult judgments to make about questions of who was entitled to treatment, open discussion amongst my team of some seventy people, who have a variety of perspectives, would resolve these issues sensibly and responsibly. After all, they more than anybody were sympathetic to the needs of couples with fertility problems, and they had considerable experience – more than any ethics committee or indeed, for that matter, the HFEA.

I was astonished, and horrified, at their reaction. Most of the team, particularly the junior members, were not only hostile to the idea of treating Sheila, but felt almost threatened by the idea. They did not seem to want to consider the issue rationally. Some of their arguments seemed completely extraneous and irrelevant. 'What if the press got hold of the news that we are treating an HIV positive patient?' was one frequently voiced objection, as if the rights and wrongs of a person's treatment could be seen in terms of good, or bad, publicity for the hospital. Others, female members of staff, said that thinking as mothers they couldn't allow the unit to bring a child into the world who might die, or whose mother might die. This understandable and emotional response became less easy to justify when it was pointed out that we treated couples with genetic diseases in their families who were taking these decisions. Other women we treat might die of pre-existing diseases whose therapy – for example, for breast cancer – had made them sterile. It was also increasingly clear, that much to our shame, some of my team, whom I have always thought of as an extended family, were actually frightened at the idea of treating a patient who was HIV positive for fear, in some entirely irrational way, that they might contract this disease themselves. As the meeting continued, it became obvious that we were not going to be able to have a logical or rational discussion and the meeting became increasingly heated. It was the first time I fully appreciated the appalling stigma that people suffered through having contracted the AIDS virus, and the horrifying fear that even some responsible health care professionals had of this disease. Eventually the meeting closed with no consensus, although some of the older people present clearly felt that we should be treating this couple.

I came away from that meeting very depressed indeed. I was increasingly convinced that this couple deserved and required this treatment. I was also sure that, if my team's irrational reaction was typical, they would not find it possible to get their IVF elsewhere. My depression was partly the thought of having let down my patients, but also a strong feeling that my team, a group of people who I admired, had let me down. I have a very special affection for the team of people with whom I work, and huge respect for their judgment and expertise. Previously, I had always believed that when difficult decisions needed to be taken, the difficulties should be shared and we should, in a democratic way, arrive at the best solutions. I left the meeting having learnt that clinical decisions about who should have treatment could not be decided by committee or by some kind of democratic decision. Whether the decision is taken within a close-knit team like my own or by, for example, some purchasing authority or the HFEA that could not intimately understand the needs of a particular patient in question, collective decisions must be more likely to be fallible. I learnt that there were certain medical decisions where a relatively autocratic decision was needed. I resolved that I should continue to do my utmost to arrange treatment for Sheila and Alan, though it was many months – after individual discussions privately with members of the team – before we were able to take her through a treatment cycle. The treatment failed, and a year later Sheila remains fit and well, and still wanting a child. I certainly intend to try further treatment, if circumstances remain the same.

Just this week, when writing this chapter, I came across a rather silly article in one of the Sunday newspapers. In it the director of one of Britain's more fashionable and expensive private IVF clinics was apparently quoted, in an entirely different context, as saying: 'If we think a couple would make perfectly good parents, we wouldn't refuse to treat them'. To me, this shallow comment, if true, sums up so much of what is wrong with the way we currently deploy some of our medical resources, particularly in the field of infertility which is not a condition perceived as life-threatening. It is the concept that anybody, fertility expert or lay person, can actually decide whether or not a couple would make 'perfectly good parents' – not only that, but presume to do so on the basis of possibly a 20-minute consultation in the highly artificial environment of an IVF clinic. I have no idea whether Sheila with her HIV infection, or indeed any of my patients, will make good parents. In fact, I am not certain whether I would qualify for that accolade myself. What troubles me most about this arbitrary process, whereby we impose our values on other people – often perhaps those who are less articulate, knowledgeable, or well provided than ourselves – is that we are in a position to do so simply because they are suffering from a disease process. No other free member of society is vetted before he or she decides that they want to try for a baby.

Of course people do not have a right to have a child. However, in a society which considers that its citizens should have proper medical care provided for and regulated by the State, those citizens also have a right to fair and equable treatment. That does not always happen in this country at the moment. Whether or not infertile couples get competent, sensitive investigation, whether or not they receive the standard of treatment they have a right to expect, whether or not they pay varying amounts of money for IVF depends on too many irrational, essentially arbitrary and unfair decisions. We live in a relatively rich and well-organised society which repeatedly states its belief in the value of family. Our society, therefore, needs to understand that the resources which we already have available should be better distributed to those seeking to produce and promote their family.

Chapter Two

Male Infertility

The commonest cause of male infertility is a poor sperm count. The actual number of sperm produced may in itself be low. Alternatively the quality of the sperm, either their ability to move or develop normally, may be at fault. As I mentioned in my introduction, most adult males produce an ejaculate of around 5 millilitres (about a teaspoonful) and usually there will be at least 20 million sperm in each millilitre of seminal fluid – the average being around 60 million. In most fit males at least 40% of the sperm will be motile – that is to say, capable of swimming reasonably fast in a roughly straight line. Normal sperm are also capable of increasing their speed, becoming hypermotile, when coming close to the egg, to facilitate their penetration. When a man is subfertile, the number of sperm that are produced will be abnormal, having an abnormal head or two tails, or some other feature incompatible with normal fertilis-ation for the most part.

Generally there are two basic causes of a poor sperm count. The testicle may not be producing enough sperm, or sperm of the right quality. Rather infrequently, the testicle is so badly damaged that it produces no sperm at all – so called testicular failure. Alternatively, the pipes leading from the testis are damaged. As this tubing pro-vides an important environment for the sperm to under-go their final growth process – maturation – damage to it can cause immature sperm to be produced. Severe damage leads to blockage and no sperm at all can pass. Seminal fluid is still produced from secretion from glands in the male ducts, but it contains no sperm. I have heard some male patients refer to this as 'firing blanks'.

The general causes of male infertility appear to be numerous. In the case of blocked tubing, most, but by no means all, of this damage worldwide is caused by sexually transmitted diseases such as gonorrhoea, or by tuberculosis. The causes of testicular malfunction are more complex and, for the most part, we do not really understand why the testicles are not producing sufficient sperm in the majority of infertile men. Certainly, environmental factors may play a part, and it is said that stress, fatigue and ill-health all contribute to a poor sperm count. Some environmental poisons, for example, insecticides, heavy metals such as lead, and certain drugs such as cannabis or alcohol, undoubtedly depress testicular function in some men and probably account for some male subfertility. However, the only well-defined poisonous activity which has clearly been shown to depress sperm production is heavy cigarette smoking. Even here, the evidence is not absolute because it is true certainly that the majority of men who smoke are perfectly fertile.

There has been considerable recent publicity given to the idea that possibly throughout the world, and certainly in Europe, men have been becoming progressively less fertile. The evidence for this is said to be that sperm counts done in various fertility laboratories around the world have shown a progressive decline in the last fifty years. In essence, it has been suggested that we are doing something to our environment which is poisoning it. Chemicals such as insecticides used for intensive farming, or some persistent detergents used in industrial processes (which, it has been suggested, may have female hormone-like properties), which leak out into our water supply had been blamed both by some scientists and by government sources. The more strident environmentalists, who seldom look at data carefully and objectively, have called for a halt in the use of these chemicals. The more strident journalists, who do not check the data at all, suggest that the human race is dying out, with its

Julia and Martin

Martin Sayers seemingly has everything: money, a good job in the City, a mansion, horses, and a wife of eight years' standing – Julia. But he is infertile.

Though Julia agrees that impotent men are seen as 'weedy' 'wimps' – Martin flatly disagrees. 'Let's face it, Tom Cruise has the same problem as I do and half the women in the world want to sleep with him.' Martin polishes his machismo as coach of a local under-elevens football team.

For the four IVF attempts, Martin produced semen in the hope his sperm would fertilise eggs, but because his sperm were so few in number and moving sluggishly, we had sperm ready from a donor. These were held in reserve in case there was no chance of fertilisation with Martin's sperm. Before agreeing to this, Martin and Julia were given extensive advice and counselling and were made fully aware of the ethical and emotional implications of using donated sperm.

After repeated IVF failure, they remained desperate. At the fourth attempt, Julia became pregnant. Incredibly and cruelly, in spite of all medical precautions, the waters around the baby broke after twenty-two weeks of pregnancy and her baby died.

In spite of this disaster, they wished to do everything to continue. By this time the new treatment of male infertility, direct injection of sperm into the egg (intracytoplasmic sperm injection or ICSI), had been developed. Martin and Julia were keen to try it and to improve his chance of producing the 'best' sperm. Martin got into training: he took up regular running and limited his alcohol intake.

Ironically, at this stage, it was Julia's biology which twisted fate. As sometimes happens after repeated IVF attempts, she started to respond very poorly to the drugs needed to stimulate her ovaries. To make matters worse, she developed a uterine cyst which necessitated temporary suspension of treatment. When, finally, the couple was able to be reinstated on the programme, Julia's womb lining remained thin and her ovaries produced only four eggs despite heavy stimulation. However, Martin's efforts paid off and his sperm – though vastly and visibly inferior to donor samples – were good enough for ICSI. After sperm injection, one of the eggs fertilised, but the uterine lining grew so badly we felt it was extremely unlikely she could become pregnant. We therefore decided to freeze this single embryo in the hope we could transfer it later, after stimulating her uterus to produce a more receptive lining.

Embryo transfer was done several months later, after repeated treatment to get her uterus in the best condition. Julia became pregnant, only to miscarry after a few weeks. Julia's and Martin's situation typifies the problems which occur when several factors in both partners contribute to the infertility.

genitalia shrivelling up and its sperm production being poisoned in its own waste. In fact, there is very little serious evidence at all that men are less fertile now than they used to be. There are several serious flaws in the data. They compare sperm samples from men who turned up for fertility treatment fifty years ago with men now, and it is highly probable that the demography of fertility clinics has changed considerably. The men of the 1940s and 50s, who are acting as the base population for comparison, were likely to be from a different background both socially and medically. It is highly probable that they were therefore not comparable with men who are now attending infertility clinics. Fifty years ago, methods of sperm counting were totally different. (Sperm counts have always been notoriously inaccurate and, to a large extent, still are.) In the 1950s, the optical quality of most laboratory microscopes was inferior, the way seminal fluid was prepared for assessment was less stringent, and the conditions under which sperm were sampled were all quite different. Therefore to make accurate comparisons with sperm assessed by current techniques is extremely difficult, if not impossible. But even if we were clearly able to prove that sperm counts in many men are lower than they used to be, this is not good evidence that men are necessarily less fertile.

Until quite recently, there was little in the way of satisfactory treatment for men with poor sperm counts. It is true that blocked ducts can be operated upon and the blocked parts removed, but few surgeons seem to have bothered to develop proper expertise to do this. The diameter of the epididymis, the main, very coiled tube leading from the testis where most blockages occur, is not more than about 0.2 millimetres in diameter. That is to say it is finer in external diameter than the cotton used to sew buttons onto a shirt. To make surgery more difficult, it has a consistency not unlike wet tissue paper, making it extraordinarily difficult to repair, necessitating microscopic surgery so that the surgeon has a magnified picture of what he is seeing. Moreover, special material and instruments are needed. It may sound shocking to say this, but it is true that very few urological surgeons doing male infertility surgery have gone to serious lengths to get themselves trained to do this work in the most effective way. In fact, to this day, most surgeons operating on infertile men still use the unaided naked eye. Consequently, it is hardly surprising that results from this kind of surgery are appallingly poor. In recent years, with the advent of IVF and the increasing acceptability of donor insemination, these operations have come to be perceived as old-fashioned because there are alternatives which require less skill, or training of a different kind. This is a pity because it limits the options of infertile men who might be highly suitable for microsurgery done properly.

Most male infertility is caused by failure of sperm production from the testis itself. Over the years numerous remedies have been offered to the unfortunate men who have poor sperm counts. There are at least 200 different drugs which have been used. It is axiomatic that if there are 200 different remedies in the pharmacopoeia for a particular condition, none of them works except in rare circumstances. Some of these drugs are quite powerful hormones, often causing quite unpleasant side-effects such as impotence or loss of libido. Infertile men have also been subjected to operations to remove veins around the testicle (so called varicocoeles); again, the evidence that this is of much value is largely dubious except in uncommon circumstances. Men with poor sperm counts have also been in receipt of a huge amount of home-spun and largely unhelpful advice. This includes advice on bathing the scrotum twice daily in cold, preferably iced, water. (This advice may sound unbelievable but I have recently seen it repeated in a 'quality' national daily newspaper, in an article stating that all men are becoming less fertile because of contamination in the environment.) There is also the common, and mistaken, idea that men who are subfertile should not have intercourse too often, 'for fear of weakening the sperm count'. There is not the slightest evidence that reducing sexual activity helps. Advice about stress, driving a vehicle and altering one's occupation is equally prevalent, and equally irrational.

There have always been three other alternatives for infertile males. Firstly, providing that enough sperm were capable of being produced, washing the seminal fluid to remove débris and dead sperm, and then inseminating the fluid into his partner's vagina (artificial insemination by husband or AIH), had modest success rates, of between 4–9%, depending on how bad the sperm quality was. The second was, of course, adoption but adopting a baby is, as is described elsewhere in this book (page 65), excessively difficult. Thirdly, there was the possibility of artificial insemination by donor (AID – nowadays more usually referred to as donor insemination or DI). Donor insemination, like adoption, is not really a treatment for infertility, but more a way of having a child by alternative means. DI is not always quite as successful as might be thought. Donated sperm has to be frozen to accommodate a quarantine period, preferably of three to six months whilst tests are done to ensure the donor is free of serious illnesses, such as viral hepatitis. The freeze/thawing procedure undoubtedly reduces the fertility of the sperm, and few clinics get much better than about 8–10% chance of a pregnancy each month with donor sperm. Many healthy women, with nothing wrong at all, repeatedly fail to conceive with multiple insemination attempts.

IVF has radically changed treatment of the infertile male. The ability to wash what sperm are available after purifying the seminal fluid in the laboratory and then place the best sperm in close contact with the egg, freshly collected from the ovary, has been a major advance. In most good clinics, IVF for male infertility has a roughly 30% chance of success with each cycle attempt. Until recently, the main restriction has been on the number of sperm available, conventional IVF requiring around 100,000 sperm to give a reliable chance of fertilising an egg. As most infertile men produce perhaps ten times this number of sperm, it can be seen that IVF has been a huge step forward.

However, the really dramatic progress has been with sperm microinjection. It is now possible to inject single sperm directly into the egg using a powerful microscope equipped with micromanipulators. Early work in this field started many years ago in animal eggs, and it was found possible to fertilise mice eggs fairly reliably by injecting single sperm into them. A sperm was sucked up into an extraordinarily fine glass needle, which was passed through the outer coat of the egg, the zona pellucida, and then through directly into the substance of the egg, its cytoplasm. However, at that time, this was considered much too dangerous for human use. It was thought that injecting sperm directly into the cytoplasm of the egg might damage the genetic material inside it, the chromosomes. It was also felt that in an infertile male there might be a severe risk of injecting a genetically abnormal sperm, which had not been filtered out and discarded by the natural protective processes.

In the late 1980s, Dr Simon Fishel, then working in Nottingham, proposed an alternative to direct injection of sperm into the centre of the egg. He suggested that it might be simpler to inject sperm just under the zona, the outer shell, from where the sperm might penetrate the cytoplasm itself. His argument was based on the understanding that amongst men with not very motile sperm, many had sufficient movement to enter the egg, providing the hard outer shell was first penetrated. He also felt that it would be safer to assist fertilisation in this way because there would be no disruption of the egg itself and no penetration of its cytoplasm and hence a risk to the chromosomes. Moreover, he suggested that there would still be some degree of selection of sperm as it would be unlikely that very damaged sperm would be able to enter the cytoplasm. Dr Fishel's suggestions produced an extraordinary amount of often quite virulent criticism. Dr Jack Cohen, a well-known physiologist who has spent much of his working life studying sperm, said publicly and very vigorously that he was deeply concerned about the technique. He felt there were real dangers associated with it because injection overrode the natural selection process. Dr Cohen was particularly anxious that abnormal babies might be produced.

All the disquiet made it impossible for Dr Fishel to pioneer sub-zonal sperm injection (SUZI) in Britain. In spite of repeated representations, the then licensing authority (the regulatory authority which preceded the HFEA) refused Dr Fishel a licence to conduct a pilot study on human patients. He decided, because he felt there was sufficient evidence of the technique's safety in animals, to look round for a unit overseas which would allow him to continue his research. A unit in Rome greeted Dr Fishel with open arms, and he proceeded to treat a number of infertile Italian couples. On this occasion, at least, Italy's lack of any serious regulation in this area worked very much to the advantage of some of its population when a number of despairing couples gave birth to completely normal babies. Soon after, English patients who could afford the journey flocked to Rome. Within months of Dr Fishel publishing his impressive results, various doctors around the world safely repeated them and more pregnancies were generated. Still Dr Fishel was prohibited from gaining a licence to carry on the work in Britain, and in consequence a number of couples who would probably have benefited from the technique did not have children. Age now prevents some of them from having any serious chance of producing a baby.

The whole episode raises interesting issues. Amongst them is the question of whether regulatory bodies are justified in preventing the development of a treatment, when they have no evidence that it is dangerous, and when seriously-minded individuals themselves, after proper informed consent, decide that they would like to take the risks involved. My own view is that regulatory organisations, such as the HFEA, do need to pay more regard to the principle of respecting the autonomy of the people who are actually suffering from these problems.

With more research, Dr Fishel's pioneering work was superseded. SUZI gave way to an even better technique, in fact the method that was originally pioneered years earlier in mice. This method, intracytoplasmic sperm injection (or ICSI for short) has now replaced SUZI almost entirely. This in no way diminishes Dr Fishel's important contribution, because he certainly paved the way internationally for the acceptance of the more advanced technique. As it happens, ICSI is also subjected to some fairly ludicrous regulation by the HFEA – but more of that later.

ICSI was largely developed in Belgium by Professor André van Steirteghem and his colleagues. It is possibly one of the greatest advances made in infertility treatment and certainly the most important development for the treatment of infertile males. If a man can produce a single sperm, then ICSI may be able to help. Moreover, the sperm do not need to be able to move at all and do not need to be mature. Couples whose only previous chance for a baby was via DI, with no genetic relationship to the 'adopting' father, are now able to consider this treatment. Because the sperm do not need to be mature, even men who have total blockage of the epididymis – or, indeed, any part of the male tubing from the testes – can be helped by sucking sperm directly from the blocked tubing, or indeed from the testicle itself. Remarkably, the sperm injection can be with sperm which are virtually dead, or bizarrely, from the genital tract of a recently dead corpse.

There are still concerns about the safety of ICSI; for one thing selection of sperm cannot be other than random. Consequently, there is the theoretical risk that an abnormal sperm might be injected, with dire genetic consequences. However, the evidence so far strongly suggests that if an abnormal sperm fertilises an egg, no viable embryo is made and consequently there seems no chance of pregnancy. Also, in order to pick up a sperm for injection into the egg, the sperm's movement needs to be slowed right down. This is done partly by cooling the sperm, but more usually by immersing it in an extremely viscous liquid. This liquid, which is very thick, prevents the sperm's tail from beating vigorously. Nearly all units use a solution called PVP, and there is concern that this could be very toxic. However, in Europe alone, well over one thousand babies have been born after ICSI using this compound, and there has been no evidence at all of any increase in numbers of abnormal births. Babies born after ICSI seem to have no more chance of mal-formation than do babies born after natural conception or after routine IVF.

ICSI requires exquisite technique to work. The human egg is only 100 microns in diameter, thinner than a human hair and invisible to the naked eye. When it is initially collected from the ovary, it is surrounded by very sticky helper cells. These cells, which come from the follicle in which the egg develops, are crucial to the egg's final development. By totally enveloping it, they are able to provide essential nutrients and remove waste products from the egg. In all, the egg is surrounded by about 2–3 million of these cells, and all of them have to be removed under the microscope before sperm injection can be started. Once the egg is cleaned, it has to be held rigidly

Male Infertility

under the microscope so that its outer zona can be penetrated. The microscope under which the egg is viewed, all the instruments needed, and the egg in its culture solution are mounted on a very heavy table, usually made of marble and weighing anything up to a quarter of a ton. This is to isolate the egg from any vibration. In the early days when we started this work experimentally, we found that a lorry driving past the laboratory, perhaps 30 metres away from it, could cause huge vibration, particularly if discharging its load. Even placing the table on a concrete floor did not completely isolate external movements, and we had to mount the table on air-filled rubber balls (rather like squash balls) before we could kill external vibration sufficiently.

The instruments, too, have very precise requirements. They are made from glass tubing which is drawn out to an extremely fine diameter after heating. The heating is done by an electrical filament (rather like an electric light bulb filament, but without the surrounding glass) and various mechanical devices have been invented (some much more effective than others) to ensure even traction when drawing out these fine pipettes. Two types of pipette are mainly needed. The first is the fine holding pipette, about 0.04 millimetre across which has a smooth end and to which gentle suction is applied, to hold the egg immovably. The injection pipette is very much finer and its internal diameter ideally should be no wider than the sperm head which is to be picked up in it. This holds the thrashing sperm tail immobilised. Remarkably for such a small instrument, the tip of the pipette has to have a fine bevel on it so that it can penetrate the egg and cause minimal disruption to its cytoplasm. These instruments, which are all 'home-made' in the laboratory, are so delicate that, if waved around too vigorously in the air, they can snap. The laboratory staff spend many hours making them, and a good amount of glass pipetting has to be discarded before getting a single instrument which is 'right'.

Obviously such fine instruments cannot be man-
oeuvred by the unassisted hand, and micromanipulators
are needed. These devices are geared to transmit hand
movements at perhaps one hundredth of the initial
movement. Thus if the gear stick of a micromanipulator
is moved in a particular direction for 10 centimetres, the
tip of the instrument which is held in it will move
1 millimetre. Movements inside the pipette are transmitted by tubing attached to the pipette. A fine syringe
with a screw barrel can transmit tiny amounts of
traction. The whole set-up is quite expensive; we spent
about £40,000 on our first injection set-up, including the
closed circuit television system which is fairly essential if
an accurate record of the procedure is to be kept and
different members of the team are to be taught how to
improve their technique.

A major problem with sperm injection is that it is
extremely laborious – and labour intensive. It needs
very special dedication from a highly committed person
to get it up and running. In our unit, we owe a huge
debt of thanks to Dr Hock Chieng, the staff member
doing most of the ICSI. Hock is one of the most keen
and eager of the staff, and meticulous about getting the
mechanics of things right. When he gets very excited
about what he is doing, he seems to jump up and down,
and his voice goes a little bit squeaky – he is the perfect
Piglet in our forest. He became so committed to sperm
injection that he used to sleep overnight on the
premises and, often for the best part of a week, he would
never be more than 20 yards from his laboratory. This
dedication enabled him to beocme highly proficient at
sperm injection quite quickly, but it did have some
quite funny consequences. Our first ICSI laboratory was
deliberately established at the Royal Masonic Hospital
where we had plenty of space to experiment. The hospital, being private, is very quiet, particularly at night.
The IVF laboratories are in a separate wing of the

hospital which is very deserted and isolated and, of course, securely locked and alarmed against any possible intruders. Night porters in the hospital, not knowing of Hock's presence there, would see lights going on and off on the unit at perhaps one or two in the morning. Hock being so short could never be seen. On one occasion, I was telephoned at home at 4.30 a.m. by the hospital switchboard, who were convinced there were ghosts on the unit. They had seen lights go on and off, and had seen Hock's laboratory gown waving at the window briefly, but the alarms never went off. It was some time before I could persuade them that this was just the diminutive Dr Hock, doing one of his night-long stints.

Of course, sperm injection has, as its main indication, male infertility. However, even when the sperm are completely healthy, not all the eggs fertilise. On average, about 62% of eggs will fertilise during a typical IVF cycle. If the eggs are slightly immature or if their outer zona is hardened for some reason (it is thought that the eggs of older women may be particularly liable to this kind of hardening), then fertilisation rates may be a good deal lower than 60%. It is also true that some women have eggs which are prone to polyspermy – that is to say their eggs become fertilised with more than one sperm simultaneously. Such polyspermic eggs have three or more sets of chromosomes (instead of the normal pairs) and therefore are not compatible with normal life. Many IVF workers have suggested that sperm injection, by ensuring fertilisation of the egg with one sperm only, would be a widely useful technique to improve all IVF attempts. Usually, even when the sperm are subfertile, we get up to 80% of the eggs fertilised, so the extra fertilisation would presumably give more embryos and improve success rates. This theory has yet to be proved, but it is certainly clear that ICSI is an extremely powerful tool, whose full potential has not yet been developed.

One of the current difficulties of developing ICSI in Britain seems to me to be the excessively bureaucratic regulatory body, the HFEA. We have already seen how Dr Fishel's work, which eventually benefited many overseas patients before being allowed in the UK, was prohibited by the then regulatory authority. Since the development of ICSI, the HFEA has seen fit to place numerous restrictions on its use. Some are clearly sensible, others seem relatively pointless and almost arbitrary. The general effect of these will be to limit the number of units doing ICSI, making it a more privileged and expensive treatment. Currently, it is insisting on a number of limitations to ICSI, which are not necessarily in every patient's interest. For example, a recent directive sent to all IVF units carrying out the treatment rules that doctors may not, at the same time, transfer to the uterus a mixture of embryos produced by ICSI and those fertilised by routine IVF. The express purpose of this ruling is to ensure that the Authority can collect pure data, knowing that any clinical outcome is related to the embryos that were transferred. However, laudable though the desire for the collection of data undoubtedly is, this ruling will not be in the interests of some patients who may wish to avoid absolute commitment to the relatively new treatment of ICSI. Many women with infertile partners, whose ovaries yield a large number of eggs, may want to split the yield. They may prefer to try to have some eggs fertilised naturally, leaving the remainder to ICSI. In the possible event of having one egg from each batch fertilised, they would be less likely to get pregnant, simply because of this ruling. All this is undoubtedly not in a patient's best interest. If I wanted to collect data about ICSI, I would be required to apply to my local ethics committee and then ensure that the patient signed his or her written consent. The HFEA can do this without a patient's consent at all. This might be justified if there was the slightest evidence that ICSI was a damaging or dangerous procedure, but there is no such evidence. Moreover, the HFEA is being inconsistent. With embryo freezing there is evidence of a potential risk, yet the regulatory body cannot be persuaded to collect data on embryo freezing.

Until the development of ICSI, things were fairly bleak. Most couples faced with a really poor sperm count gave up. A few lucky ones were able to adopt a baby, but less than 1,000 babies each year are available for adoption in Britain. Few couples, except those with rare and exceptional strength, are able to take on a child who is much older, and who is likely to have come from a disturbed or damaged background. Moreover, partly because of the rarity of babies for adoption and the prevalence of infertility, agencies – mostly local government authorities – undertaking to supervise adoption have been able to become increasingly strict about who is eligible. In recent years, prospective adopting couples have often been put off adopting by the incredibly invasive vetting procedure. It is not at all easy for a distressed infertile couple, whose dignity has already been threatened by the nature of their fertility problem, to answer personal intimate questions about their family life and attitudes, particularly when the assessor may be a young unmarried social worker with less experience of life than the people he or she is vetting as suitable to look after a child. Moreover, nearly all adoption authorities unfairly insist that prospective couples considering adoption firmly indicate that they have given up (and will continue to relinquish) all infertility treatment. This is a particularly difficult undertaking today, when so many major advances are being made in fertility treatment, and when there is so much publicity given to them.

I see the decision to adopt a child as a particularly mature one. It is interesting to consider why infertility is such a serious condition for some people. I have already alluded to the severe distress it causes, but it is quite difficult to understand quite why it is such an injury. I believe that the answer is because it affects a deep-seated aspect of our being. One aspect of being human is a recognition of being mortal. We are faced with that mortality at various stages of our lives, for example, at the time of the death of our parents. Feeding from the Tree of Knowledge, but not from the Tree of Life, has given us a clear vision of our fragility. No matter what we achieve in life, whether we become rich, powerful or famous, our contribution is ephemeral, and we are rapidly forgotten. Even if we win a Nobel Prize or the National Lottery, or we become a Cabinet Minister, within a very short time we are forgotten. Admittedly a very few people are given the special gifts of Mozart, Shakespeare or Breughel, and their memory is assured. Yet every one of us ordinary people can have immortality in the children we produce, who bear our same genetic message, to a large extent unique, and many of our attributes and our aspirations. This is why I believe that almost certainly the worst form of bereavement a person can suffer is the loss of a child. After this, perhaps in some cases, is loss of the ability to have a child. The adopting couple then are doing something both mature and noble, in furthering the next generation and bringing up with love a child that is not theirs.

Even if adoption were widely available, and carried no risks, it would not be for every couple with severe male infertility. Donor insemination is an alternative that, increasingly, many couples come to accept with readiness. It has all the advantages of adoption, with the added benefit that the child is at least genetically related in part to its parents. Moreover, it allows nurture of a baby from pregnancy and birth with a fuller influence throughout all its formative time. It is also relatively easier to obtain.

Until relatively recently, donor insemination carried an undoubted stigma. The stigma was largely because any child born as a result of DI was technically illegitimate.

Moreover, though seldom challenged in the law courts, DI children were not entitled to inherit from their parenting father's estate. This stigma is now receding, not least because of changes in British law regarding the status of children born by DI. Until 1990, an adoptive father putting his name as the genetic father on the birth certificate of a DI child was committing a form of perjury. However, as far I am aware, no man doing this has ever been pursued through the courts. The 1990 Act of Parliament ensured that the father whose name appeared on the birth certificate was at least a legal parent. The Human Fertilisation and Embryology Act also ensured that children, born as a result of DI, could if they wish trace their genetic father after growing up. The 1990 Act made provision for a register of all sperm donors, and ensured that all units doing DI kept an adequate confidential register of the real genetic parentage of any offspring born.

A great deal has been written about what it feels to be a recipient of donated sperm. Parliament held agonised debates about the issue in 1990 and, by law now, anybody being offered donor insemination must also be offered counselling. The law protects the recipient and, to a degree, any child born as a result of DI. The donor is not in such a protected position. Perhaps because donating sperm is seen as a trivial thing (one wonders if sexist attitudes are prevailing), indeed pleasurable momentarily for the donor, donors are not taken seriously, providing they are healthy. Most sperm donors in Britain have traditionally been university students (most frequently studying medicine) because access to such potential donors is easy. However, for a great many reasons they are not particularly suitable.

Most university students will not be of proved fertility, being mostly unmarried, and indeed unready for a permanent relationship. A routine sperm count, as we have already seen, may not be particularly good proof of fertility. Indeed, it is well known in some DI clinics that certain donors are not at all fertile even though their counts seem adequate. Not only are they not of proved fertility, but their genetic 'risk' is even more vague. There is no clear way of establishing, by routine screening procedures, that a given donor is free of genes which are likely to give rise to a serious inherited disease in any offspring. The best that can be done is to get a reasonably comprehensive genetic history of the donor's family. This, though, will by no means reliably ensure that the donor is free of a particular genetic trait. In general, the donor's own children would be the best, if inadequate, screen, and university students who are donors do not generally have children. Another serious objection to students being donors is that they are quite likely to be amongst the most promiscuous of men. Young, free of serious attachment, still probably exploring their sexuality, they are at considerable risk of contracting sexually transmitted infections. Even though sperm may be held in quarantine, and though donors are checked routinely for HIV and hepatitis, there is no guarantee that immediately after checking, they do not contract an infection from a casual partner. That this actually happens, I have little doubt. I have encountered several female patients who have contracted pelvic inflammatory disease during courses of DI. In each of these cases, an initial laparoscopy before DI showed completely normal tubes and ovaries, so it is extremely likely that the subsequent damage was a result of exposure to infected seminal fluid.

Another source of concern about any student donor is that he may not be the most suitable genetic parent for a given recipient couple. Great concern is shown by most recipient couples to ensure the best possible 'match'. That is to say, most parents want a child who at least resembles the male partner. Virtually all DI clinics record a donor's racial background, hair colour, eye colour, physique etc., but play less attention to what is probably as, if not more, important. Using medical students as donors, often achievers in a particular academic field, may not be the most suitable match for the varying intellectual backgrounds of the recipients. This kind of consideration is, in my experience, never even discussed by clinics undertaking this work.

Perhaps the biggest source of concern is how a donor may feel after giving away his unique genetic material. Not enough serious research has been done on this issue, although Professor Robert Snowden of Exeter University has made extremely important observations. Donors are not required to be counselled beforehand. They may not have considered that they probably will not be informed whether or not they have produced children as a result of their act of donation. They may well not have thought of how a future partner might feel, knowing that somewhere in the background are step-children. They almost certainly will not have thought of all the implications of one of their future children either knowing or not knowing that they have a half-brother or -sister. The risks of an unknown half-brother of half-sister meeting an unrecognised sibling and marrying them has been a great criticism of DI. It is this fear which has resulted in a relatively arbitrary ruling that no donor should have his semen used more than ten times. It has been widely agreed that there should be a restriction on the number of children from a particular donor, but I know of no absolute figure enshrined in law. In fact the risk of consanguinity is likely to be truly remote, but it does exist. It is this reason, above all, why orthodox Jews, for example, will generally not countenance donor insemination. But in truth, whilst the risk of consanguinity is minuscule, the question of having an unknown extended family is never discussed. Yet the concept cuts across many of the concerns about family that most human societies have.

Professor Snowden's research clearly shows that some donors, long after the act of donation, deeply regret having given semen. They regret not knowing whether or not they have had children, and feel threatened to think that somewhere in the wider society, they may have offspring whom they do not know, and for whom they are not responsible.

But the donor's position is now even slightly more serious. Since the change in British law, the donor's name is recorded in confidential records which must be held by the clinic, and to which the HFEA has access. Children born as a result of donation will have the right to approach the HFEA to get non-identifying information about their genetic parent. They will be able to find out his walk of life, and something of the sort of person he was. They will not be able to obtain any information which could lead to their father being identifiable. However, there is always the uneasy feeling for donors that perhaps this law could be changed retrospectively, and that although they are anonymous at present they could find an unexpected child or children turning up on their doorstep in future. There is no doubt that this concern will continue to make it harder to recruit suitable sperm donors.

Of course, the keeping of a donor register is only of value if recipient families are open about the act of donation. In many families, DI is kept a close regarded secret, even from the resulting child. Indeed, it is my impression that probably at least two-thirds of parents accepting DI do not inform any close relative, including their child, about the true genetic parentage. This strongly suggests that, amongst other things, there is still a deep feeling of shame and guilt associated with donor sperm and with the blurring of family relationships that can result. It also suggests a perception that there are dangers in telling a child of his true origins.Whatever feelings the issue may give rise to, there is certainly quite a paradox here. The State now demands that DI units register the donor of semen so that the child can potentially trace some information about his or her father; however, neither the State, nor the doctors in the clinic, can force a couple to divulge information that they do not wish to be disclosed. The State also demands that couples be offered counselling by clinics, but it would be interesting to know what the 'take up' rate of counselling is. No one can insist that a couple undergoes counselling. Of course, when there is any counselling to prospective parents, counsellors will invariably emphasise the risks involved in keeping acts of donation secret.

Whilst, at first, to many couples considering the treatment, secrecy seems the obvious and least damaging way of dealing with donor insemination, it is undoubtedly of high risk to all concerned. Firstly, keeping a secret of such magnitude causes serious stress and may place great strain on a relationship. This stress may well increase rather than diminish with time, as the 'adopted' child grows up. Moreover, family secrets have a habit of coming to the surface. There is the strong possibility that a child may find out at the worst possible time. This may be at puberty, during an act of serious rebellion, when one parent breaks the news in anger. Possibly the secret may surface if the parents split up. Nearly 40% of married couples do not remain married to each other in our society. If and when a break occurs, all relationships may be subject to acrimony and anger, and a secretly produced child is at terrible risk then. Children can occasionally find out that they are not genetically related to their father at other times, too. A child who is ill with leukaemia, or possibly renal failure, and whose only hope of life and health is a transplant from a related donor may find it extraordinary that his apparent father is of totally the wrong tissue type.

Many of the other issues associated with sperm donation are similar to those concerned with egg donation. They include whether donors should be paid, and whether donors who are in some way genetically related to the recipient parents should be encouraged or restricted.

In IVF, one of the biggest and most common problems is that of the infertile man with a variable sperm count. His seminal fluid may just be fertile enough on a good day, but not good enough to fertilise his wife's eggs on a bad day. In such cases ICSI may not be applicable or appropriate, and many units offer IVF with the husband's sperm, but with donor sperm held ready-thawed as a 'back-up'. In principle, donor back-up used carefully and wisely is a valuable adjunct. Problems arise, however, if a couple is not advised of this possibility until the last moment, when it is suddenly discovered that the husband's semen is of poor quality. To offer donor sperm at the last minute, perhaps even on the day of egg collection, is quite wrong, but it does occasionally happen in less well-run clinics. It is an offer which, though well meaning, can be disastrous if not introduced well in advance with full information and counselling.

Another practice which fortunately is now rather falling into disrepute (though I gather it does take place in some establishments – particularly in some IVF clinics in the USA) is the mixing of the infertile husband's sperm with donated sperm from a fertile donor. The idea here is to give the husband the feeling that the child may be genetically his own – because it will not be clear which sperm actually fertilised the egg. This is a form of deceit and seems quite wrong. Thereafter, parents may look at their child and wonder whether or not this child really is genetically theirs. The action of mixing sperm, and the fact that the recipients are giving permission for this, also suggests that the principles, difficulties and problems associated with DI have not been fully accepted. It seems to me that couples pursuing this course of action are probably not at all ready for any kind of commitment which involves donated material from another individual.

Genetic engineering may change all this technology in time. In three or four decades, people may well look back and think how crude were our attempts to alleviate male infertility. In the future, it is very probable that scientists will be able to reprogramme the testis to make entirely new sperm, for example, in men who have severe testicular problems. In time we may be able to culture germ cells – the primitive cells from the embryo which go on to produce sperm in men and eggs in women – from human embryos. These cells could then be injected into the testicle, where they would repopulate it. Once in the testicle they would undergo further division until totally new sperm were formed. Even though these sperm would grow in the recipient, genetically they would be unrelated to him.

This notion, that a man could be treated to produce sperm genetically unrelated to him in his own testicle, is, to say the least, extraordinarily disturbing. From there it might seem a relatively short step to genetically engineer such sperm so that they have certain specific character-isitcs, maybe even tailor-made to the recipient's request. It is perhaps all too easy to hide behind the notion that because all this is impossible at present, it will continue to be so. In 1499, Leonardo da Vinci was sitting in Milan, designing his ornithopter (the heavier-than-air machine), drawings of which can be viewed in the Science Museum in Kensington. Nobody believed that this could fly; no doubt the Duke of Milan's courtiers had much fun at Leonardo's expense. But they might have acted very differently had they been able to glimpse for a second into the future, and see Italian Air Traffic Control's maps of flight paths in and out of Milan International Airport. We cannot afford to be sceptical about the future; we rather have to prepare for all its possibilities.

Chapter Three

Egg Donation

When a patient's ovaries cannot produce any eggs, the possibility of receiving eggs from a donor may be suggested by the doctors. A suitable donor is found and her ovaries are stimulated with drugs, and any eggs collected. These are then fertilised with the patient's husband's sperm and the resulting embryos can be transferred to the recipient's uterus. Most women who cannot produce eggs are also not producing female hormones in sufficient quantity. Therefore, before the embryo transfer, they are given extra oestrogen to stimulate the uterus just enough to help any embryo implant. Once the patient becomes pregnant, the developing pregnancy will itself provide sufficient hormone to ensure safe antenatal development.

Egg donation is, at one level, one of the great success stories of IVF. It offers an unprecedented opportunity to women whose ovaries have failed. Previously, their only chance of a child was adoption and the experience of pregnancy and delivery could not be theirs. One advantage over adoption is that many couples feel that if they receive a donated egg, then any child born will at least be related genetically to one partner. Rather surprisingly, egg donation cycles are actually more likely to be successful than routine IVF treatments. A single IVF cycle, using a woman's own eggs, has on average only about a 15% chance of resulting in the birth of a live baby. If donor eggs are used, success rates can be often doubled or even tripled. The figures opposite give the British national success rate, reported by the HFEA in 1994. They are an average, being the combined figures from all clinics doing this treatment in the UK. It is worth comparing these figures with those for routine, conventional IVF on page 29.

	Cycles treated	Pregnant %	Live birth %	Miscarried %
Under 25	8	37.5	37.5	0
25–29	55	16.4	7.3	25
30–34	134	27.6	20.9	24
35–39	128	25.8	24.2	6
40–44	142	16.9	12.7	25
Over 45	79	25.3	17.7	30

It is clear why egg donation cycles are more successful than when a patient's own eggs are used. Egg donors are young women, under the age of thirty-five and as we have seen, younger women are much more fertile. This is largely to do with the quality of the eggs stored in their ovaries. As a woman ages, more of her eggs seem to develop genetic defects when they mature. Eggs from younger women fertilise more readily and produce embryos which are much more likely to implant. It is interesting that miscarriage is also slightly less common after egg donation (compare the table above with the one on page 154). The reason for the better outlook when donated eggs are used is not entirely certain, but may in part be due to changes in the hormonal environment in the body that occur with age, and partly due to the long-term effects of gradual exposure to poisons and other contaminants that we all experience from our external environment. It is also possible that continued exposure to naturally produced background radiation may affect the quality of eggs in some older women. Another important reason why egg donation is more successful is that, during a routine IVF cycle, a woman is given large doses of drugs to stimulate her ovaries. This certainly has the desired effect of forcing the ovaries to produce as many eggs as possible, but will have adverse effects on other organs, such as the uterus. Vigorous ovarian stimulation results in a large number of follicles being matured, but also stimulates the ovaries to produce huge amounts of oestrogen, the female hormone. During a typical IVF cycle, the ovaries may produce five to ten times the normal amount of oestrogen. This gets into the blood stream and is carried to the uterus where it has an effect on the uterine lining which is very responsive to oestrogen. This stimulus may result in the uterine lining becoming too thick and less able to allow the embryo to implant. In an egg donation cycle, the recipient of the fertilised eggs is not exposed to excess oestrogen, but is simply given precisely the right amount of this hormone to make her uterine lining develop optimally. It is also possible that the huge doses of stimulatory drugs themselves may have a bad effect on the uterus. A recipient of donor eggs therefore is more likely to have her uterine lining in a more natural state and this makes implantation more probable.

Egg donation is needed quite frequently because there are many situations when a woman cannot produce eggs of her own. We have already seen how the menopause results in the ovaries becoming depleted of all eggs. Quite frequently, women can have a premature menopause. This devastating condition, which can occur in very young women (in their twenties, or even occasionally as a teenager), is caused by the ovaries running out of eggs too soon in life. The reason why this condition is relatively common is not at all clear. It is possible that, due to some congenital problem, most of these young women started life with too few eggs in their ovaries. It is equally possible that in some cases they may have developed some unknown internal condition resulting in large numbers of their eggs being destroyed before or just after puberty.

In some cases, a premature menopause is caused by a clearly diagnosable genetic defect, most usually an abnormality in a woman's chromosomes. One typical example of this is Turner's syndrome. This is one of the commonest chromosomal disorders, and occurs when a girl is born with only one X chromosome instead of the normal pair. Turner's syndrome, in its most severe form, results in the ovaries being completely absent. However, quite frequently, the ovaries are formed, but there are either no eggs inside the ovaries or very few. Girls with Turner's syndrome also tend to be very short in height and do not menstruate. Because their ovaries produce very little oestrogen, they start to experience all the effects of the menopause twenty or thirty years early. In order to prevent these effects (loss of bone tissue, heart disease and general aging) they need to take extra oestrogen as a drug, so-called hormone replacement therapy.

Many women start life with normal ovaries but they become very badly damaged as a result of diseases developed during adult life. Young women who suffer from very large ovarian cysts and who need many repeated operations to remove them can end up with very few eggs in their damaged ovaries. The most important disease which causes this problem is endometriosis. This scarring condition is caused by deposits of the lining tissue normally found inside the uterus. When it is abnormally situated – for example, inside the ovaries – an endometrial deposit can bleed with each menstrual period and scar tissue and cysts are formed. The cyst presses on the surrounding ovarian tissue; the healthy ovarian tissue degenerates and eggs are lost. Very severe inflammation of the ovaries, perhaps associated with chronic infection of the fallopian tubes and abscess formation in the pelvis, may also cause depletion of the egg supply. This can follow venereal diseases such as gonorrhoea, but there are many other infections such as tuberculosis which can have a similar effect.

Some women, particularly those women in their late thirties or early forties, become what are called 'poor responders'. These women, for reasons which are not at all well understood, stop being able to produce eggs, even when stimulated by the powerful drugs given during IVF. Other women with a variety of hormonal conditions which result in a failure to ovulate may also be only likely to get pregnant if they receive an egg donation.

Some women (like Rebecca, whose plight is described on page 144) develop cancer at a young age. There are a number of cancers which may affect young women. Perhaps the most important is chronic leukaemia. Until recent years, diagnosis of this terrible condition was generally a death sentence. Nowadays it is possible to treat leukaemia very effectively and so most young people who are treated survive. Treatment involves replacement of the bone marrow after giving massive doses of X-rays. One of the most important and unwanted side-effects of the irradiation is the sterilisation of the patient; massive irradiation generally kills all the eggs in the ovaries. In a tiny percentage of these women, the ovaries may recover somewhat after irradiation and menstrual periods and ovulation may resume; most, however, are made menopausal. Other highly curable cancers which occur in young women are Hodgkin's disease, cancer of the lymphatics and breast cancer. Sufferers from these diseases are increasingly seeking egg donation after their cancer is cured.

Another reason why some women seek egg donation is because a serious genetic disease is carried in their family. Sometimes there is no effective gene probe for the defect, which means it cannot be detected during a pregnancy. This means, of course, that women who would normally consider a termination of a pregnancy, knowing that the baby suffers from an hereditary defect, cannot do so. Such women may seek a donated egg from an individual who is free of this hereditary disease as being the simplest way to conceive a healthy child.

In view of all the reasons for seeking donated eggs, it is clear that there are many women who seek this kind of IVF treatment. Unfortunately for them, there are very few women who are ready to donate eggs. Study of the table

Egg Donation

on page 154 shows that only 546 egg donation cycles were done in Britain last year. I calculate that there must be at least 20,000 women who would benefit from this treatment, but there is a huge shortage of suitable donors at the present time. There are many reasons for this.

An egg donor has to undergo considerable medical treatment. She will need to take the fertility drugs which are usually given to infertile women during an IVF cycle, to make her ovaries produce as many eggs as possible. These drugs have numerous side-effects which an infertile woman will fairly happily tolerate because she knows that taking these drugs will give her the only chance of a pregnancy. It is entirely different for an altruistic donor. Fertility drugs can often make people feel rather unwell, or depressed. Abdominal bloating and tenderness are common. Hot flushes and headaches are quite frequent. Very often taking these drugs disrupts the menstrual cycle, causing irregular bleeding for several months after treatment with them has stopped. Taking these drugs may also temporarily disrupt one's sex life. But there are two more serious side-effects, which are of more concern.

During treatment with the drugs, the potential egg donor will need to have very careful, regular supervision. She will need to have daily ultrasound assessment, and many hospitals also prefer recipients of fertility drugs to have repeated blood samples in addition to ultrasound testing. Regular attendance at hospital for all this is pretty daunting, especially for a young woman who may be bringing up a young family, or who is required to be at work by a certain time in the morning.

Even with close, regular supervision, fertility drugs can cause hyperstimulation. This condition occurs when the ovaries over-respond by producing too many follicles containing eggs. The ovaries swell up and instead of being their normal size (about that of a plum) they can become as large as a football. Associated with this are changes in the blood which can make it more sticky and likely to clot. Hyperstimulation at its most serious can even be fatal, and certainly one infertile woman in the UK has died from its consequences. Of course one does not want to exaggerate these risks because with proper care they are usually preventable; nevertheless things can go wrong even with the most responsible medical team. There is no doubt that it is perfectly reasonable for a fully informed, consenting patient to undergo these risks in the hope of having the benefit of her own child. However, there are ethical problems about allowing another person to run this risk when she can receive no personal benefit. There is also some evidence, certainly not proved, which suggests that fertility drugs can possibly induce ovarian cancer many years after they have been taken. Although there is very little evidence for this, there are undoubted ethical concerns about causing any risk of this sort to a person who does not need to experience it.

Egg donors also need an operation to remove the eggs from their ovaries. Admittedly egg collection is a relatively minor operation, but it can result in post-operative pain and, as with any anaesthetic procedure, there are always slight risks of accidents, such as internal bleeding. Of course, an operation like egg collection may be much more likely to just make a person feel rather unwell, but this too will stop the motivation of some potential donors.

Egg donors are also required to undergo screening. Before going into a donor programme, they will need to have a number of blood tests and possibly genetic screening to make certain they are healthy. They will certainly have to have screening for viral infections such as hepatitis or HIV, and many women will be put off being donors because of this. The implications of finding out that one has a fatal virus like HIV are extremely serious, and many women are put off this screening, even if there is absolutely no reason for them to consider themselves at risk.

If all this medicalisation were not enough of a disincentive, there are the concerns that the donor of genetic material will always have. They have already been discussed in relation to sperm donation; they are, however, more critical for egg donors because most egg donors will have to be of proved fertility (that is, having already had a child) and are usually married. Consequently they will need to think very carefully about the implications of having children whom they do not know, and their existing children from their marital relationship possibly having half-brothers or half-sisters about whom they can know nothing.

The Human Fertilisation and Embryology Act emphasises the need for IVF units to provide a counselling service. No area of reproductive medicine raises as many important issues requiring patients to get careful counselling as does egg donation. In the past, most of the counselling emphasis has been devoted to the potential recipient of donated eggs or sperm. The recipient, after all, has to bring up a child, for whom she will be responsible for life. But donors are placed in a potentially vulnerable position, particularly if they know the recipient, or are related to them. Whether donation is done anonymously, or whether a donor offers to give her eggs to a particular infertile couple known to her, she needs extensive and sensitive counselling. In Britain the track record is good in this respect, but I am unconvinced that donors worldwide always get the best care. The advantages to clinics in finding donors to supply their desperate infertile patients are considerable. The commercialisation of IVF is widespread in many developed countries and the risks of donors being exploited is certainly present. In view of all these concerns and constraints, it is hardly surprising that there are far fewer potential donors than recipients. Given these problems, where do most egg donors come from?

There are basically five potential sources of donated eggs at present. Generally, probably the commonest source is young women undergoing IVF because they themselves are infertile. There are obvious advantages to this arrangement. These women need to take the drugs concerned for their own treatment and have to have the operation to collect eggs anyway. They are therefore not undergoing any increased physical risk. Moreover, the monitoring – the ultrasound and blood tests – are no extra problem for them because they need this for their own treatment. Because they are infertile themselves, they will often be very strongly motivated to help other women who are suffering many of the same emotions.

To my mind, however, the IVF patient is a very unsatisfactory source of donated eggs. The main problem is due to the fact that, at present, there is no way of storing eggs safely. Eggs have to be exposed to sperm within a few hours of being collected from the ovaries. This means that the IVF patient who donates some of her eggs to another woman may find that the recipient of her eggs gets pregnant, but the eggs she retains for her own treatment, may not fertilise – or alternatively do not produce viable embryos. In effect she has gone through an expensive and demanding treatment for a condition which is causing her extreme sadness, entirely for the sole benefit of another individual. This seems to me to be entirely unethical. One way of getting round this problem is to offer the infertile patient who is prepared to donate some eggs free IVF treatment. There are a number of clinics that do this in different countries. But this risks making matters even worse because it seems there may be a serious risk of coercion. Under these kind of circumstances, a donor may take excessively damaging or unnecessary risks out of sheer desperation or because of inability to pay her way for her own treatment. I have even seen cases where women, producing a larger than expected crop of eggs, have been repeatedly badgered by unscrupulous doctors to consider egg donation. It is even possible that such doctors, because of the commercial advantages to them, might consider stimulating the ovaries too vigorously just to ensure that extra eggs may be available. The needs of the desperate and sometimes demanding young menopausal patient should never persuade doctors to lower proper ethical standards. It is the duty of doctors doing IVF to protect all those under their care, and to ensure that the decisions they may take even voluntarily do not subsequently cause them grief.

A second source of egg donors is women coming into hospital for a variety of gynaecological procedures. Women undergoing sterilisation, for example, may be thought to be ideal candidates as donors. They will have completed childbearing and will also, of course, have proved their fertility. Very often they are very ready to volunteer this service, without first being approached. Women coming into hospital for hysterectomy may be another source of donated eggs. However, there are problems with such donors as well. They are usually likely to be of relatively advanced reproductive age as few women undergo hysterectomy under the age of forty, or sterilisation under the age of thirty-five. This means that they may be donating eggs which carry an unacceptable risk of a chromosomal defect, such as Down's syndrome. Another problem is that the fertility drugs that they need to take to stimulate their ovaries may make the routine operation for which they are coming into hospital a bit more complicated. The ovaries will undoubtedly be enlarged and the blood supply much richer than in the unstimulated state. There is therefore more likelihood of sudden bleeding during surgery. There are also more likely to be postoperative complications – possibly including the potentially serious one of clots in the veins, or venous thrombosis. Venous thrombosis can lead to clots on the lungs – in rare circumstances a fatal event and, although this is not at all likely, doing an incidental egg collection after ovarian stimulation certainly raises the risk. For all these reasons very few egg donations have come from gynaecological patients.

Close relatives of the infertile woman needing donated eggs – perhaps a sister – are frequently motivated to think of offering their eggs. Very serious issues are raised by this. Even if such an act of donation is done with complete love and consent at the time, feelings between the various people involved may well change later. The indebtedness that such a valuable and extraordinary gift produces may well result in different emotions such as resentment and conflict many years afterwards. If such an act of donation is done openly, problems may arise as any resulting child grows up. The child may perceive three parents and may possibly feel more attracted to his or her genetic mother than to his 'adopting' mother. This could cause serious family difficulties and jealousies, particularly if the adopting parents are not getting on together. There is evidence to suggest that a child in this situation may feel extremely confused and that this in time could lead to serious psychological problems. It is also possible that such an act of donation could result in a change of relationship between the genetic father and the donating genetic mother, leading to marital difficulties in possibly two marriages. If on the other such an act of donation is undertaken in secret, with for example only the parents knowing about it, then there is always a risk of the resulting child discovering that the mother with whom it has identified is not genetically related. If this discovery happens, for example, during vulnerable adolescence or when a parental marriage is breaking down, the damage to the child could be extremely serious.

A fourth source of donated eggs is close friends. Here,

possibly, matters are not quite so fraught as they are when close relatives offer their eggs. Nonetheless, similar issues of secrecy and problems of confidentiality are raised. There is always the thought that the donating, genetic mother may continue to feel a close identity with any child that is produced. It is important for doctors undertaking this work to remember that approximately 40% of marriages in this country break up, mostly quite unpredictably. It may be that, in the event of growing unhappiness between adopting parents, a genetic mother might feel a powerful urge to interfere in the nurture of a child suffering as a result of an unhappy parental relationship.

One of the potentially very serious concerns about using a friend or a relative as a donor is the worry about whose responsibility it is should a genetically damaged child be born. Although I have never seen this happen, eventually an act of egg donation will result in a baby being born with a chromosomal defect, most likely Down's syndrome. The egg would, of course, have been damaged before being donated and the genetic 'responsibility' will have been the genetic mother's. An unresolved question that is raised is who takes responsibility for the care of the child, should he or she be rejected by the bearing mother. Legally, of course, there is no doubt that the bearing mother is fully responsible for any child born to her after egg donation. Nevertheless, the emotional implications between donor and recipient after such an event are clearly very worrying.

One of the problems about assessing the risks arising from egg donation from either close friends or relatives is that there is, as yet, no firm information about the long-term outcome after such arrangements. Egg donation is a very new field. The only parallel treatment is sperm donation, but outcome after sperm donation is a poor model. This is because it is very much easier to give sperm than it is to give eggs. Also, it is quite possible that women feel differently about donating their genetic material. Clearly this is an important area for research, but it will be many years before there is any substantial information which will help us decide how serious all these rather theoretical risks are.

Some clinics have thought of an ingenious way round the problems of confidentiality or lack of anonymity between related donors and recipients, or between friends who give their eggs. When patients needing egg donation request treatment, the clinic may suggest that the patient brings her own donor – either a relative or a friend, or possibly a sympathetic woman who the patient recruits. Such patients are then 'paired' with other patients who have similarly brought a donor with them. Each donor is then able to give eggs anonymously to the paired recipient. There are considerable problems, however, with this approach. Firstly, it puts an extra burden on egg recipients who have to 'recruit' a donor. They may, privately, give incentives of possibly a financial nature to the prospective donor who is thus coerced – possibly against her better judgement – into a treatment which may cause her emotional problems. Paying donors is not legal in this country, and therefore any arrangement of this nature would have to be clandestine. Secondly, many related donors and recipients feel that they want to give or receive eggs from their relative because by doing so, they at least ensure some familial, genetic link with the child. Many donors who are relatives of infertile women find it much harder to go through egg donation if they feel that their unique genetic material is going to an unknown family. Finally, there is the serious risk to any relationship if half way through finding out how difficult and potentially traumatic being an egg donor is, a relative or friend pulls out of the arrangement and refuses to give her eggs even though she initially agreed to do so. Such situations will cause great grief to all concerned and even the strongest friendships or family relationships may be seriously damaged by this unfortunate turn of events.

For all these reasons, I feel that there are no easy solutions to egg donation. At Hammersmith, we are convinced that the best donors are undoubtedly those few altruistic members of the general public, women who are giving their eggs with no strings attached. They are prepared to go through the risk and inconvenience of egg donation because of a strong sense of sympathy with infertile women. However, such donors are not easy to recruit, particularly if clinics take a responsible attitude towards them and take great care not to encourage them to do something they may possibly regret later. These donors generally hear about the plight of women who need donated eggs from press publicity. Very often, a young woman with a premature menopause is televised, and a wave of sympathy encourages women to write in, offering their eggs. It is interesting to see how few of these well-meaning women turn out ultimately to be suitable donors.

The results of our first television appeal for donors give a very good idea of the difficulties in finding suitable, anonymous donors. After one television programme, we had 403 women write in offering their eggs. My team laboriously contacted them all, in itself quite a lengthy procedure. Ninety-four of them had changed their mind after having written to us. Another eighty-seven basically had gynaecological or fertility problems of their own which they really wanted to discuss with a sympathetic doctor. Very often they felt that they were not getting the correct treatment from their GP or local hospital. Then 131 women pulled out of offering egg donation as it gradually became apparent to them that the procedure involved them in much more medical treatment than they had imagined. Twenty-seven did not relish the idea of the detailed screening that would be needed, particularly for the AIDS virus. This left just sixty-four women who appeared to show continued interest in being an egg donor. Of these, only twenty-two continued to attend hospital for counselling and the various tests that were needed – just 5% of the original number who showed interest. A number of these women were unsuitable as donors for a variety of reasons and eventually, from the original 403, we were left with eight women who remained committed and were entirely suitable donors. This is a huge amount of work for so few donors, each of whom will only be able to go through one or possibly two cycles of stimulation at best.

One ethical issue that has recently been raised is the question of whether egg donors should be entitled to payment. The HFEA stipulated originally that there should be no payments made for donated eggs and at the time this seemed highly reasonable. The idea of a trade in eggs is abhorrent to many people, reducing what should be perhaps an act of altruism into treating genetic material as a kind of commodity. Moreover, it was widely felt that this could lead to exploitation of poor people, their possibly being led to give eggs to those that could afford to have a baby. Consequently, the HFEA only allowed payment of modest travel expenses to donors. During the year, I became increasingly convinced that this restriction was too severe. One donor travelled a distance of over 700 miles backwards and forwards for scanning during her donation cycle. She handed in expenses of £42, costed at six pence for each mile travelled in her small car. I felt very unhappy about this because her time travelling alone was over twenty hours and this seemed to be ludicrous recompense for her extraordinary act of kindness to a person who was totally unknown to her. I think that it would be reasonable to offer such women two or three hundred pounds – not a vast sum, and certainly it seems to me not a sum which would lead to serious exploitation. Since this issue was raised in the press, the HFEA has relented somewhat and appears to be about to agree to modest payments to egg donors.

People from different walks of life, and people with different ethnic origins may have very different attitudes to egg donation. We have found it difficult to recruit donors for African women or those coming from a Caribbean background. Whether this is because they have a different perception of family or possibly genetic relationships is hard to say. Women coming from the Asian subcontinent often seem able to recruit donors from their own close family, but seem to shun the idea of giving eggs to an anonymous, unrelated individual. Jews have problems with both donated sperm and eggs. Amongst orthodox Jews, egg donation is almost unknown in this country. Jewish law is very concerned that children should know who their parents are, not least because there is concern that a half-brother or -sister might unwittingly marry a sibling and thus commit incest. Some Jewish religious authorities have suggested getting around this problem by accepting eggs from non-Jewish women. As the bearing mother is Jewish, the child would automatically be Jewish. As such a child would normally only marry another Jew, these authorities have ruled the possibility of unwittingly committing incest is thus eliminated.

The shortage of egg donors from the general population is not likely to change. In our unit, after extensive screening, we recruit no more than six to ten donors each year. Each may, at most, contribute two treatment cycles i.e. two lots of eggs. With luck, a good donor cycle will yield enough eggs to treat two, or at most, three patients. As we see at least 200 couples a year who would benefit from the receipt of donor eggs, it is obvious that there can be no way that we can meet the huge demand that exists.

There are, however, considerable possibilities for the future of egg donation, and there are grounds for considerable optimism that the plight of young menopausal women may be improved. The most likely advance is unquestionably research into freezing eggs. If human eggs could be stored in liquid nitrogen, they could be fertilised later for transfer to a menopausal woman. This overcomes the main objection to using 'spare eggs' from patients undergoing IVF. If frozen storage was perfected, then spare eggs could be held until it was clear that the donor's treatment had worked and she had safely become pregnant and possibly delivered. She could then give approval for her eggs to be used by another woman, without risk of exploitation or any coercion. Egg freezing at present is still regarded as too risky for clinical use. Although there have been two births in the world after freezing of human eggs, there is currently considerable concern about the dangers. As we have seen in Chapter One, Resources, embryo freezing is widely used and, oddly to my mind, few scientists or doctors have any worries about it. My own view is that in the long-term, egg freezing may actually be safer. Once sufficient animal experimental work has been done to find a safe way of carrying it out, it would have great advantages over embryo freezing. At present, the problem is that freezing of eggs is thought possibly to risk damage to the chromosomes and damage to the tiny structures inside the egg which ensure its normal subsequent development. This damage largely depends on the speed at which freezing is done, and the chemical protectants used to prevent ice-crystal formation disrupting the cell. Consequently, with further research these problems could almost certainly be solved.

Widespread use of egg freezing and storage would mean that there would be less need to keep embryos 'on ice'. Frozen embryos are a kind of hostage to the fortune of their parents. Should something happen to one or both

Egg Donation

of them, the disposal of embryos is always going to raise problems. Unfertilised eggs carry much less moral status and their disposal would therefore presumably be easier, less subject to litigation, for example, in the event of divorce. Egg freezing could also in the long run be safer. This is because after thawing, a frozen embryo is more or less immediately transferred to the uterus – there cannot be significant delay to observe it growing to see if it is developing normally. A thawed egg automatically will undergo a test of its normality when fertilisation and subsequent embryo growth is seen over several days. If the freeze/thaw process had caused damage, fertilisation would be very unlikely to occur, as would cell division. It is probable that in the next two years, human egg freezing will become an established procedure, as it is gradually being researched successfully in animals. There will then be more hope for those women who need donor eggs.

There are other even more remarkable advances on the way, which are relevant to the plight of women needing eggs. Approximately two years ago, extraordinarily extensive press coverage was given to the idea that eggs suitable for donation might be retrieved from fetal ovaries. This was simply a gentle suggestion made by an eminent scientist, Professor Roger Gosden, then working in Edinburgh. He was not researching this subject in humans and, perfectly properly, he was running the idea in front of an ethics committee to see what their reaction might be. As eggs are formed in the ovary well before birth and are held there in a state of arrest pending adulthood, Dr Gosden had argued that this might just possibly be a good source of eggs for the treatment of women who were unfortunately experiencing a premature menopause. The fetal ovary is smaller than the adult ovary, and yet contains ten times more eggs (about five million) than does the ovary of a mature woman. Here then was a huge concentration of eggs, potentially ready for harvest providing methods could be developed for maturing these immature eggs outside the body. Not perhaps surprisingly, there was a wave of press and public reaction. Religious organisations – particular those with strong views about abortion – were almost incandescent with anger that doctors could apparently consider taking eggs from dead babies or, worse still, from aborted fetuses. The HFEA rapidly – possibly too rapidly and without enough preparation – started a public consultation process to see what various organisations and groups with an interest in the subject might feel. It probably would have been better to have firmly stated that this was simply a research idea, and like many scientific ideas was completely unfeasible at present. It should perhaps have pointed out that, even with intensive research, it would have been at least ten years before such an idea would have a chance – if at all – of coming to fruition. Because the discussion was not put in this context, the story gained credibility in the newspapers, and one or two doctors who were not actively involved in any of this research went on television to discuss the work; I felt strongly they should not have talked about the subject in such an irresponsible manner. Of course, this provided a further stimulus to public 'outrage', although I suspect, like in many matters of this kind, most men and women in Britain did not seriously regard the subject as a grave threat to the moral fabric of British society. At the time, as my car was not working, I conducted a straw poll amongst London cab drivers (always an interesting and informed source). I never detected much serious outrage amongst them, nor amongst pregnant women and other fertile and infertile couples in my clinics. Nevertheless, the story gained momentum and it culminated in a rapidly produced Parliamentary Bill, introduced by the trenchant Dame Jill Knight, calling for a ban on research involving human fetal ovaries. Reprehensively, the then

Egg Donation

Secretary of State for Health, Mrs Virginia Bottomley, supported the Bill, and fetal ovarian research was banned. I write 'reprehensively' because it would have been far better for Mrs Bottomley to have waited to hear the deliberations of her own appointed expert regulatory authority, the HFEA. To introduce hastily legislation (which was completely unnecessary, seeing as nobody was even seriously considering doing such research) was to ensure inadequate discussion and reflection. It also undermined the standing of the HFEA, which was surely unwise.

It is perhaps worthwhile briefly discussing why so many people had such anxiety about fetal egg donation. Understandably, there was concern that a child might be born to find that his 'mother' was actually an aborted fetus, possibly terminated for some social reason. People also expressed abhorrence at the idea of taking germ cells from a dead baby in this way. There was also concern that women might be prepared to deliberately enter into a transaction whereby they aborted their fetus to give its eggs for commercial purposes. I am not sure how the anti-abortionists thought that such immoral women would be able to ensure that their aborted fetus was a little girl before embarking on a pregnancy. Most people discussing the subject ignored the fact that eggs might be retrieved from miscarried fetuses, where there had been no interference to produce a baby's death.

But what was really surprising about the whole debate – which was generally not at a very high level – was the fact that nearly everybody discussing the issue and pontificating about it, doctors included, failed to recognise or point out that it might be equally feasible to take eggs from adult ovaries. Each square millimetre of adult ovary contains many hundreds of eggs. Take a tiny biopsy from an adult ovary, no bigger than a pin-head, and after maturing these in culture they could possibly be used for subsequent donation.

There are many advantages to working with adult ovarian tissue. Firstly, it is possible to obtain totally informed consent from the donating woman. Secondly, in an aborted or miscarried fetus, the ovarian tissue is usually extraordinarily difficult to identify. Moreover, as with any corpse, there is the risk of contamination and the likelihood of getting tissue which has already degenerated. There would be no problem of this kind when using adult ovarian tissue, taken in a sterile manner by permission during some incidental gynaecological operation, for example. Thirdly, of course, in the adult ovary there will already have been some degree of maturation, and any eggs may be likely to be easier to culture. Moreover, the ovary of an adult donor will have already produced eggs and the donor can be shown to be fully fertile and free of any obvious genetic defect.

At Hammersmith Hospital we have started to try to recover fertile eggs from small pieces of donated ovarian tissue. Pieces of ovary are obtained with consent from women undergoing operations for a variety of gynaecological reasons. Microscopic follicles are taken from the tiny ovarian pieces. The follicles are then cultured in an oven at body temperature, and the culture fluid in which they are bathed is repeatedly dosed with hormones. Nutrients, such as sugars, and substances known to encourage growth of cells are added. We have already managed to grow invisible follicles to a few millimetres in size. These are the first steps that have been successfully taken in maturing adult human eggs in a culture dish. It is likely that within the next five to ten years we will be able to grow fertile human eggs in vitro in this way. Once we can do that, the problems of egg donation will be largely resolved.

There are other colossal advantages to working with small pieces of ovary in this way. Pieces of ovary can be safely stored by freezing them in liquid nitrogen.

Egg Donation

Professor Gosden and his colleague Professor David Baird from Edinburgh's Reproductive Biology Unit have already successfully frozen pieces of sheep ovary. To demonstrate that the ovarian tissue was still viable and able to release its eggs, they did the following experiment. Some weeks after the freezing, the ovarian slivers were thawed and the scientists then transplanted the ovarian pieces back into sterilised sheep. The ovarian slices subsequently released their eggs, and the sheep successfully delivered live lambs. I think it only a matter of time before we are able to freeze-store human ovary in this way.

I believe that this work, together with the ability to culture human eggs from pieces of donated human ovary, paves the way for the most important advance in the whole of human reproduction. Within the next decade, we shall not only have solved the problem of egg donation by this approach, we shall have solved many of the difficulties involved in IVF procedures. The ability to mature eggs from small pieces of ovary in the laboratory will lead to the simplification of in vitro fertilisation, and to a huge reduction of its total cost. In ten years' time, an infertile women will come to the infertility clinic and under a quick local anaesthetic, with a procedure lasting less than ten minutes, two microscopic pieces of her ovary will be quickly removed via a needle inserted through the vagina. The pieces will be frozen and stored in liquid nitrogen, where they could remain almost indefinitely without deterioration. When the woman is ready to have a baby, the ovarian biopsies will be thawed, the follicles harvested and placed in culture dishes. They will then be dosed with drugs to bring the eggs to maturity. All the woman will need to do will be to bring a sample of her husband's semen for the fertilisation of the eggs. When embryos are formed, she will simply return for a two-minute procedure – the embryo transfer. She will need to take no expensive and debilitating drugs. She will need no hormone tests or frequent attendance for daily ultrasound. The medical costs will be about one-quarter of what they are currently for IVF, and hundreds of pounds will additionally be saved because stimulatory drugs will no longer be needed. The savings to the NHS will be huge and there will be far less excuse not to provide this treatment on a wider basis. It is also clear that the emotional strain on the infertile will be diminished because there will be fewer uncertainties and less medical intervention.

Culturing stored eggs in the laboratory in this way also has important implications for women who may be made menopausal by cancer treatment. Before undergoing chemotherapy or radiation, ovarian tissue could be stored in liquid nitrogen. Once the cancer is fully cured and the patient ready to have a baby, eggs could be matured and placed into the uterus after IVF.

There is one other fascinating implication of this extraordinary technology. In future, ovarian storage in this way could be used as a form of family planning. It would certainly get over the problem of the fertility of women reducing with age. A university student stores pieces of ovarian tissue whilst taking her law degree. She then studies for the bar and enters chambers. Years later, she takes silk and becomes a senior barrister. When her financial situation is secure and her marital relationship stable, she can return for her eggs to be fertilised. Even though she is now in her forties, her eggs are as fertile as they were twenty years earlier, and becoming pregnant should not present a problem.

Egg donation, then, has led to an extraordinary expansion of IVF treatment. This expansion is still leading us into areas which are not fully charted. It widens the application of IVF to many women who previously would have no chance of giving birth. It even offers the potential of manipulating and controlling our reproduction in ways which we certainly did not even consider only four or five years ago. It also carries great human responsibilities. It has led to a re-evaluation of motherhood, and threatens our conventional notion of family relationships. It implies a moral necessity to protect those women who, mostly for very altruistic reasons, act as donors of what is possibly the most valuable gift that anyone can offer. Research and clinical practice in the field of egg donation should be clear examples of how medical science must work for the benefit of the human relationships which this field was designed to promote.

Chapter Four

Embryo Research and Testing for Genetic Defects

G enetic desease is truly almost the last great unsolved medical problem. If you are born with a disease which is purely genetic in origin, the chances are almost certain that you will die as a consequence of it. Genetic disease is extraordinarily common. One in every fifty babies born will have a major birth defect, one in 200 will have a chromosomal defect. Over 100,000 women are admitted to hospital with miscarriages each year, and the vast majority of this loss of life is caused by a genetic problem in the fetus. One-quarter of all children in hospital are suffering with what is primarily a genetically-determined illness. One in eight adults in hospital have a genetic component to their disease and there is, to some extent, a genetic basis for cancer, heart disease, diabetes and some psychiatric disorders.

Diseases which are purely genetic in origin are generally in one of three categories. The first are the single-gene defects caused by an abnormality in the DNA, the blueprint held in the cell which determines the proteins our bodies make and hence our physical and some mental characteristics. Usually, single-gene defects occur as a result of a misprint in the letters of the DNA at one point somewhere along its length. There are about 5,000 different diseases caused by single-gene defects. The commonest in Britain is cystic fibrosis, which causes severe lung damage and defects in the digestive organs. Another very important disease, because it kills about 250,000 babies around the world each year, is ß-thalassaemia. This is a severe blood disorder causing a fatal form of anaemia.

The genes are placed next to each other on long strings of DNA, the chromosomes. The chromosomes are in the nucleus of the cell. Each gene can be regarded as a

Embryo Research and Testing for Genetic Defects

paragraph of information – like an entry in an encyclopaedia, each chromosome a complete volume and the whole DNA (or genome) as the complete encyclopaedia of life. To continue the analogy, the DNA is kept in the nucleus, the bookcase if you like, in each cell. This encyclopaedia is identical in each microscopic cell in the body. Each human cell nucleus has 23 pairs of chromosomes numbered according to their size. Chromosome pair number 1 is the largest, pairs 21 and 22 the smallest. The twenty-third pair is the sex chromosomes which are partly concerned with determining a baby's sex. If our sex chromosomes are XX, we develop as female, if XY male. One of each chromosome pair is derived from the father via the sperm cell, one from the mother via the egg. Chromosomes can be damaged or absent, and this causes the second category of genetic defects, the chromosome disorders. The commonest chromosome disorder compatible with life outside the womb (most chromosome defects cause such severe abnormality that the fetus is not viable) is Down's syndrome, caused by three copies of chromosome pair 21. Another disease is Turner's syndrome (see Chapter Three, Egg Donation) and is caused by absence of one of a pair of X chromosomes; it results in a girl's ovaries being improperly formed.

The third category of pure genetic defects are the developmental abnormalities. These are not generally caused by problems in a single gene or a damaged chromosome, but rather by some adverse influence during early human development. A very good example of these are the arm and leg defects seen in thalidomide babies. The genetic damage caused by giving this drug in pregnancy resulted in failure of these limbs to develop properly. Another typical example of developmental abnormality is the congenital blindness sometimes seen in babies born after their mother contracted German measles during early pregnancy. There are a number of

Debbie S. and Chris

Debbie was twenty-seven when she first attended our clinic. She had been married to Chris for about a year when she conceived. Her little boy, Nathan, seemed reasonably well at birth, although his hair looked very abnormal. It was realised that he was seriously ill when he was four months old. Apart from showing exceptionally retarded growth, he started to have convulsions. These fits increased in number and severity and he started to show signs of slow deterioration. The paediatricians who were consulted diagnosed a rare condition called Menke's disease, which only affects boys. The gene for this hereditary disease is carried on the X chromosome, which meant that Debbie was a carrier of this severe disease and, though not affected herself, had a 50:50 chance of passing it on to any son. Any daughter would have an evens chance of being a carrier, like Debbie.

After watching her little boy gradually deteriorate, without any chance of an effective treatment, Debbie and Chris were ready to try anything. They heard of a new experimental drug treatment from the USA which they tried. For a while it seemed that Nathan's suffering lessened, but after only eighteen months of life he went into coma and died.

Debbie became pregnant again, and tests revealed it was another boy. Unfortunately, as yet there were no DNA tests for Menke's disease, so the couple had the difficult choice of aborting the pregnancy without knowing definitely whether it was affected or not. After this experience, they felt they could not go through another termination and came to us to discuss the new treatment called preimplantation diagnosis. In this treatment, IVF is done and each embryo is tested to see if it is a boy or a girl. Only female embryos are transferred to the uterus, male embryos being allowed to disintegrate in the culture dish.

IVF was tried twice. Female embryos were transferred but Debbie did not get pregnant. After much sorrow, Debbie conceived spontaneously – a boy. Further tests proved he was disease-free and, at the time of writing, her pregnancy was proceeding well.

Embryo Research and Testing for Genetic Defects

viruses, of which Rubella, the German measles virus, is the best known, which can cause severe damage to developing organs if caught by the fetus during pregnancy.

Once established, medicine can palliate but never truly cure the pure genetic diseases. Until very recently, the only way doctors could prevent some of them was by antenatal screening followed by termination of an affected pregnancy. Not all genetic diseases can be screened for during pregnancy. Moreover, different families are at risk of different genetic diseases, and the doctors have to know for which disease to screen if they are to be able to detect an affected pregnancy.

In vitro fertilisation has provided a major breakthrough in genetic disease prevention. IVF, because it provides access to the embryo before implantation in the womb, and before pregnancy commences, can now be used for embryo screening. People who carry gene defects in their family will have some affected embryos which will develop the disease. Other embryos they produce will be entirely free of the gene defect and some will merely be carriers – although not affected themselves, they can pass the genetic defect to the next generation.

The research to do this embryonic screening started at Hammersmith Hospital in 1986. IVF treatment involves stimulating the ovaries to produce as many eggs as possible. As we have seen already, it is unsafe to transfer more than two or three embryos to the uterus and there are very frequently a number of 'spare' embryos which cannot be used for a woman's immediate treatment. These spares have always presented a major ethical problem. They could be frozen for later use, but many patients do not want their embryos frozen and, in any case, embryo freezing may carry a genetic risk. They can be given to other patients, but this also raises ethical problems. They can be disposed of by destroying them. They can be given up for research, which we have found many patients greatly prefer because they feel they are contributing something in return for the technology they are using. It is these spare embryos which have provided the basis for the research on human genetic disease.

At the time we started working on genetic disorders it was well-known that before a mammal's embryo implanted, when it was about at the eight-cell stage, each cell was totipotential. Theoretically, this means that at this stage of development, each cell from an eight-cell embryo – implanted separately into the uterus – should be capable of producing an identical animal. Numerous experiments had been done – cutting sheep and mouse embryos in half and quarters, dividing the number of cells equally – and identical twins and quadruplets had been successfully produced. The animals were identical because each cell contained exactly the same DNA in its nucleus. It was therefore fairly clear to us that we could remove a single cell from a human embryo, without necessarily causing damage to it. Because the single cell that had been removed would be genetically identical to the cells left behind in the embryo, analysis of the DNA in the single cell should give precise information about the genetics of the whole embryo. Over the next four years Dr Alan Handyside, who led our research team, developed techniques for the removal (or biopsy, to give it its proper name) of single cells from spare human embryos. The biopsied embryos were not, of course, transferred to the uterus, but were grown in the laboratory for up to a week to assess the effect of biopsy. Various tests were done. We measured the rate of cell division in the embryo after the biopsy had been done, and we measured the number of cells that the embryo contained after five days following the biopsy. Both these tests are fairly sensitive indications of whether an embryo has been damaged. We also measured the metabolism of biopsied embryos to see whether they showed any chemical evidence of damage. In parallel with this work we continued gathering evidence about

Embryo Research and Testing for Genetic Defects

any damage caused to animal embryos. The evidence from various experiments in different centres including our own was that normal mice, rabbits, cows, sheep and monkeys had all been born totally healthy after embryo biopsy. This was reassuring because it confirmed that this essential part of any screening procedure was likely to be safe.

The method of biopsy was intriguing. Just as with sperm injection directly into the egg (described in Chapter Two, Male Infertility) the embryo needed to be held rigidly under a microscope with no vibration. A heavy marble table cushioned on squash balls to eliminate movement was found to be ideal. We invested in an immensely expensive set of micromanipulators without really knowing whether what we were planning was in the slightest bit feasible. The embryo to be biopsied was held by suction in a home-made flame polished glass pipette – so fine that the end of the pipette could not be seen with the naked eye. Very carefully, the smallest possible droplet of acid solution was applied to the surface of one part of the embryo, so that a borehole could be made through its outer coating, the zona pellucida. A slightly wider glass tube was now introduced through the hole and one cell carefully teased out away from the embryo. This technique was repeated endlessly until the biopsy could be made fairly swiftly, without damaging the embryo. Eventually, it was possible to do a complete biopsy in well under 5 minutes. Occasionally things went disastrously wrong, and the whole embryo would come out of the hole. Other times, we lost the tiny cell that we had painstakingly removed. The work was really only possible because of the enormous patience and gentleness that Alan Handyside showed during these stages. It was eventually found that the best time to do the biopsy was about three days after fertilisation, when the embryo had preferably no more than about eight cells. After this stage, the cells tend to form bridges between each other, and prising one cell away from the others was more difficult.

The biopsy started to go well. However, at this time nearly all IVF programmes were transferring their embryos to the uterus within one or two days of fertilisation. It was found that if embryos were kept longer than this in culture outside the body, they tended to degenerate. Because we found it technically better to delay the biopsy until the third day after fertilisation, it was obviously necessary to ensure that we could maintain the embryos in culture for that long. A number of modifications to our culture technique were instituted. We asked a number of IVF patients, who were having a routine transfer, for their permission to delay their transfer until the third day after fertilisation to test the methods. With their signed consent, we started to compare the pregnancy rates between those patients who had an embryo transferred on the second with those that had a transfer on the third day. We were pleased to find that not only did our improved culture work, but the patients having a day-three transfer actually had a slightly better chance of getting pregnant.

But the most important problem was that we still had no reliable method for genetic analysis of the cell that we removed. It was just possible to stain the chromosomes of a single cell and occasionally detect whether it had two X chromosomes, but the technique was very unreliable. The most reliable method took two weeks of laboratory work for the diagnosis. It was obvious that we did not have two weeks, because no human embryo could survive outside the body longer than three days at that time, even in the best culture conditions. Our ideal would be to remove a cell on the third day after fertilisation, make a diagnosis within eight or at most ten hours and transfer the fresh embryo to the uterus early the same evening. It was true that we might be able to freeze the embryo whilst awaiting diagnosis, but this was

Embryo Research and Testing for Genetic Defects

not an attractive option. There was real concern that freezing might do serious damage to an embryo that had a hole made in it by the biopsy.

At this time we had a young research doctor seconded to our laboratory from Northwick Park. Dr Richard Penketh was a tall gangling, very enthusiastic individual, who was always leaping about with extraordinary ideas, many of which to our great surprise worked rather well. Some of my colleagues in the lab found him a bit taxing because contents of cupboards seem to travel after an experiment. He was bursting with energy and undertook all sorts of extra jobs about the unit until, like Tigger, he was distracted by a new notion. (I still have, after nine years, half of one of the walls of my office painted a slightly odd colour.) He was convinced that it would be possible to shorten the time for genetic diagnosis as he had heard of some work suggesting this in another lab doing totally different experiments. Using embryos from mice, he started to research a chromosome stain that might, with some clever chemistry, be able to give us a diagnosis of the sex of the biopsied cell within one day.

We all realised that diagnosis of embryonic sex would be a major leap forward. There are about 300 genetic diseases which are sex-linked, nearly all of which are carried on the X chromosome by the female, but only affecting males. One of the commonest of these diseases is haemophilia. This was the terrible bleeding disease carried by female members of the Russian Royal Family, but affecting only the Tsar's son. In a sufferer, the slightest knock or bruise can produce severe internal haemorrhage, and severely affected children get bad arthritis from bleeding into the joints. Sudden haemorrhage into the brain quite frequently occurs, leading to death. Another of the most common sex-linked diseases is Duchenne muscular dystrophy, a severe progressive muscle-wasting disease which affects only boys. Most children with this disease have such muscle weakness that by the age of ten they are frequently in a wheelchair. Death occurs when the weakness becomes so profound that they are unable to breathe properly and they suffocate; alternatively they develop heart failure. Death is usual by the teenage years or, at the latest, as a very young adult. A third disease that Alan Handyside, Richard Penketh and I were interested in at this time was Lesch-Nyhan Syndrome. This also affects only boys who suffer with severe spastic changes. Because they cannot help it, they tend to self-mutilate – one child I know of bit off his tongue and chewed away his lips – the only way to prevent further damage before he eventually died was to remove all his teeth. Richard knew one woman, Julie, with this disease in her family. Julie's son, Peter, had to be continuously strapped into his wheelchair with his arms restrained. He was incontinent and needed constant all-day supervision. Julie had had no fewer than eight pregnancies – all but her one affected son had either ended in miscarriage or had been terminated because these babies were also affected with this appalling condition. We felt it would be wonderful to be able to give Julie a little girl, knowing that this child at worst could only be a carrier and not affected in the same way.

However, Richard's efforts to stain the sex chromosomes did not impress us. He was convinced he could see an incredibly vague shade of pink under the microscope with his better attempts of staining the Y chromosome. Alan and I remained rather unconvinced. At this time, however, a great advance had been made in California. The polymerase chain reaction (PCR) had been invented. This remarkable technique enables laboratory workers to make multiple copies of part of the DNA from a small number of cells. This process is called DNA amplification because from just one copy of the DNA, researchers can make over a million copies within a few hours. There is then enough DNA to measure on an analytic gel. The

Embryo Research and Testing for Genetic Defects

technique allows the analysis of the DNA to confirm that a particular genetic sequence is or is not present. It is now used for a wide range of purposes. (In the recent O.J. Simpson trial in the USA it was used to confirm that the blood stains present at the scene of the murder and on that famous glove were (or were not?) identical to Simpson's own blood.) Using PCR, DNA has also been analysed from Egyptian mummies. Its biggest and most important application is almost certainly medical rather than forensic. It is, for example, extremely helpful in trying to determine whether a baby in the uterus has a particular gene defect, and it can be used for a wide range of diagnoses of adult disorders. Its inventor, Dr Kerry Mullis, won the Nobel Prize for the invention three years ago.

Our problem was whether PCR could be used on just a single cell. This was new territory scientifically, and would require some modifications to the published technique. PCR was known to be sensitive, but there were likely to be very serious problems in getting it to work with just one molecule of DNA. We had what we thought was the perfect DNA sequence to try to identify – a sequence which only occurred on the Y chromosome, and therefore would tell us if the embryo was a male. One problem was that the PCR test was so sensitive that any contamination could mar the result. For example, a male laboratory technician clapping his hands 30 feet (9 metres) away from the tube where our embryonic cell was being placed could release one of his own skin cells and, should this float into our tube, give us a false result. It was also extremely important that when taking the biopsy we trapped no spare sperm with the cell we were removing. This, too, could give a false DNA signal.

Over many months, Alan beavered away in the laboratory trying various modifications of the PCR technique to make it still more sensitive and less liable to contamination from stray DNA. At this time we did PCR by hand. The process involved heating a small tube containing a solution with the DNA from one cell, together with the PCR reagents. Using a stop watch, every two-and-a-half minutes the temperature was raised to 93°C for two minutes, and then cooled quickly to around 61°C for one-and-a-half minutes. This process was repeated over three hours by alternately plunging the little tube into two water baths heated to precisely the right temperatures. Fairly mind-bending work, and one wet Sunday afternoon when an experiment was in progress, I took pity on Alan and lent him my portable CD player with the Neville Marriner recording of Mozart's *Marriage of Figaro*. After a bit Alan just trusted me sufficiently (or was so bored) to allow me to briefly take over, whilst he did some other pressing work in an adjoining lab. I immediately put on Shostakovitch's *Tenth Symphony* and during one of the more stirring, loud and rhythmical passages got my timing wrong, and staring at the watch in my confusion, plunged my hand (instead of just the tube) into the hotter water bath. Remarkably, when we tremulously ran the diagnostic gel to see if we had our million copies three hours later, we were able to confirm that the test had worked and we had a male cell. Fortunately, there are now machines which do PCR and the process is automated.

At this time, both Alan and I felt we were working against the clock. There was a real risk our work was about to be banned. Parliament was starting to consider the issue of embryo research. There was fierce criticism of it in the country, mostly from a small but strident group of people – the so-called 'right to life' advocates. In their carefully orchestrated campaign, they were clearly giving MPs the impression that public support for a ban on the kind of research we were doing was very great. On our side, Alan and I knew that if we could show that we could detect one of these terrible genetic disorders before

Embryo Research and Testing for Genetic Defects

pregnancy and thus prevent a woman needing to consider an abortion, we would have powerful and persuasive evidence of the need for our work. The hope clearly was to help a woman get pregnant knowing that the baby she was carrying was free of the specific defect afflicting her family.

I applied for ethical approval to biopsy a human embryo and transfer it afterwards into the uterus. The hospital ethics committee gave us permission to try the process on ten occasions and then report back. We agreed to attempt preimplantation diagnosis (which is what we called the technique) only in those women who had already lost a pregnancy or had a baby die as a result of a sex-linked disorder. We started with three very brave women. Debbie E. had had a little boy die of a sex-linked disease called adrenoleukodystrophy; Christine, whose family had had several children with a form of physical and mental retardation only affecting boys; and Julie, whose little boy with Lesch-Nyhan syndrome, was strapped in the wheelchair.

At the last moment Julie had to pull out because she had become spontaneously pregnant in spite of using contraception. Sadly, it turned out with her monstrous bad luck that this pregnancy was also an affected boy, and she eventually decided on a termination. With Debbie E. and Christine we had one false start, but then eventually got several embryos from each of them. The biopsy worked, as did the PCR. That week, on two evenings at around 8 p.m. we transferred two of their own biopsied embryos to each patient. I still recall the extraordinary feeling of trepidation I had when I transferred those embryos. My hand was steady, but my mind trembled. Even though we had by now done five laborious years of work to be as sure as possible that we could not have damaged the embryos, and even though I had complete and informed consent from both couples after full ethical approval, I did not sleep.

I do not cry particularly easily. When twelve days later the blood tests for both these wonderful patients came back positive, I have to say I cried as I told them over the telephone that their pregnancy tests were positive. I have seldom felt quite so emotional about any clinical outcome as this. Within a few weeks ultrasound confirmed normal development of the babies. Remarkably, both mothers had twins after transfer of two biopsied embryos.

We now had a race on our hands. The House of Commons was about to debate a potential ban on embryo research. A straw poll had shown that there were a large number of MPs who felt that they had to vote against our work, not necessarily out of any strong conviction that it was bad, but rather because of the pressure of a huge number of letters from supporters of the 'life' organisations. Our opponents were claiming that the research was useless, and that nobody had ever benefited from it. Some of our more vicious opponents claimed that we were telling lies when we said that we might be able to prevent some genetic diseases.

Fortunately, the Editor of *Nature* came to our aid. Not only did he rapidly publish our paper reporting our success, but he wrote a strongly supportive leader and held an influential press conference. All the daily papers and television reporters unanimously supported our work, and our two families courageously gave repeated interviews which were powerful ammunition in support of the research. But the Commons debate which followed later that week would be the watershed. Even though by now we felt we had gained increasing public support, it was not at all clear how Parliament would respond.

As this book is mostly about ethics and our relationship with moral values, it is perhaps interesting to record something of the flavour of the Parliamentary debates. The HFEA Bill had been first introduced by the

Embryo Research and Testing for Genetic Defects

Government into the Lords – a slightly unusual procedure, but done to save Parliamentary time. The debate which followed was widely agreed to show the House of Lords at its best. When embryo research had been previously debated a few years earlier, after the Warnock Commission had reported, there had been some wickedly inaccurate statements made by parliamentarians in both Houses. By this occasion, though, the Lords had informed themselves very carefully and there were some immensely impressive contributions from many peers, including the Bishops – particularly the Archbishop of York, the Chief Rabbi Lord Jakobovits and many lay peers such as Lord Carter who spoke very movingly about his own deeply felt religious values. Baroness Warnock, who had chaired the original Government Commission, gave a carefully considered speech which was appreciated by the whole House. A number of colleagues and I had made endless briefings for various peers, and I listened intently to the opinions of the peers and their interpretation of what they had seen in our work. It was a great moment when by an overwhelming majority the Lords approved of the research we were doing.

The Commons debate, leading to a free vote, which followed a few weeks later, was extraordinarily vibrant. Feelings ran intensely high. Very many MPs felt deeply about the issue – in a Private Member's motion some years earlier, a debate on the same subject had produced an overwhelming majority of more than two to one opposed to our research. Only a filibuster had prevented a ban. Virulent and deeply hurtful things had been said about our morals and our motives. Many MPs who were implacably against our work claimed we were telling lies about what we might be able to achieve. On this occasion things seemed rather better; there was no doubt that the general tenor of the Lord's debate influenced members of the Commons in producing much more temperate language than they had previously expressed on the subject. Nevertheless, all of us listening were incredibly anxious as the debate unfolded during the afternoon. I was fortunate in being allowed to sit in a 'ringside' seat, in the box under the gallery, where I could talk to MPs and could follow every nuance of what was being said. We had wonderful support from different parts of the House. Peter Thurnham, Conservative Member for Bolton NE, was a tower of strength. Although he already had a large family, he and his delightful wife had adopted a very handicapped boy. He was a trenchant supporter of any properly conducted research to prevent genetic disease. Daffyd Wigley, Plaid Cymru member for Caernarvon, had continued to devote time to help us over many years. He had lost two children with genetic disease and had made one of the most powerful speeches I had ever heard on the subject. Jo Richardson, Labour Member for Barking, had coordinated much of our Parliamentary campaign. Though crippled with arthritis and obviously in continuous pain – even standing up to catch the Speaker's eye in debate was an effort at times – she turned up for every meeting on the subject, and was always ready to give us sensible political advice between chain-smoking one of her inevitable cigarettes. Jo Richardson died in 1994 and is much missed

Sadly, some of the debate was fairly shameful. The Society for the Protection of the Unborn Child (SPUC) had run a vigorous campaign which had been part-icularly aggressive and unpleasant. At a massive rally in Westminster the week before the Commons debate some of their speakers referred to me, and doctors like me, as a Nazi experimenter. People leaving church after Sunday morning services were given misleading pamphlets telling complete untruths about our work and asked to sign Parliamentary petitions. I even met one churchgoer who had been threatened because she refused to sign. On

Embryo Research and Testing for Genetic Defects

the morning of the Commons debate, some of their members hissed at me and called me a murderer as I walked past them in the street outside Westminster tube station. The night before the debate SPUC sent each Member of Parliament a plastic model fetus in a box. This was, horrifically, the size of a twenty week pregnancy – fully formed and with all its organs carefully modelled – with a note clearly implying that this is what people like myself were experimenting upon. There was no suggestion that what we were actually doing was screening a clump of undifferentiated cells, one-tenth of the size of the full stop at the end of this sentence.

The posted plastic fetus actually misfired very badly. Most of the MPs' post was, of course, opened by young female secretaries or research assistants. A number had had recent miscarriages; some were pregnant. The shock of opening these boxes, and the campaign associated with it, produced a wave of revulsion around much of Westminster. Many friends of mine, MPs who for good moral reasons felt they should support a ban on embryo research, actually abstained on the day or voted in favour of our research. It is very interesting how a few deeply religious people, who claim the moral high ground, may be prepared to subvert the truth in order to promote their own arguments. On this occasion it was sad to see how, by corrupting their own values, they debased the important moral principles they were trying to support.

The Commons debate continued all afternoon and into the evening. From time to time a different MP came to ask me if I would like a cup of tea or something to eat. I had too much at stake and was far too nervous and miserable to think of leaving the chamber. The debate started well with a number of very positive speeches. Peter Thurnham came up to tell me that he thought that, in spite of these supportive speeches, it might be a very close decision. True the Government itself sat on the fence and was offering no lead, though Kenneth Clarke, the then Secretary of State for Health, had said that he would vote in favour of allowing our work. During the early evening, the chamber emptied and speech after speech was a long invective criticising IVF, the treatment of infertility, or the abuses of genetic engineering. By 9.30 p.m. I was in despair, and no amount of encouragement from friendly MPs could convince me that we could win, as the chamber by now was full of hostile faces and all our supporters appeared to have gone home. Just before 10 p.m. Daffyd Wigley came up. 'Don't worry,' he said, 'all our supporters are in the bar – they just don't want to listen to any more rubbish.' The vote was called and suddenly the chamber filled up. When the vote was taken, we found that we had achieved a massive majority. I have seldom experienced such elation. Members of Parliament who had grown strongly convinced of the need to support the research were hugging each other, and female MPs kissing me. All the work we had done had been vindicated. My reasons for returning to England from the USA on a much lower salary some years earlier, largely to do this work, had been justified. We were not simply evil scientists in the eyes of the public. The integrity of British science and medicine had been tested and it had been found to be valuable and laudable.

Thanks for the widespread public and Parliamentary support for this work really should go to our patients. Genetic disease in the family is often, irrationally but perhaps understandably, a cause of shame and silence. Had Debbie E. and Christine not been prepared to be very open about their family problem and tell the press exactly what had happened to them and their children, things might have been different. Their poignant stories touched a chord. There is little doubt that their bravery in being identified was crucial in helping to get this sensible legislation.

Embryo Research and Testing for Genetic Defects

Debbie was delivered of two healthy girls in the summer of 1990. Her children are just over five years old at the time of writing. Christine also had twins. Because her pregnancy was somewhat complicated, I did a Caesarean section. Very sadly indeed, one of these babies had died a few hours before birth. This was in no way connected with the genetic problem, nor was it in any way related to the embryo biopsy eight months earlier. The baby had simply outgrown its blood supply. Rebecca, her surviving daughter, is a healthy, bright five-year-old and is doing well at school. Recently Christine came back for further repeated IVF and embryo screening attempts. Sadly her ovaries just would not yield enough eggs, in spite of stimulation, and we were not able to do the procedure. Typically, Christine and her husband accepted this with their usual extraordinary good humour and fortitude.

It is perhaps at this point that I should explain why I felt then, and still feel now, that our research on embryos to improve the detection of genetic disease was justified. There are firstly the utilitarian arguments. Embryo research is clearly useful; I have already given some indication of the kind of genetic diseases that might be prevented by it. Without research on the human embryo, IVF itself could not have been developed, and most of the new treatments for male and female infertility would have been impossible. Miscarriage causes huge loss of life and great distress to women, and most miscarriages are caused by defects in the embryo. Study of the embryo will be valuable in finding how to prevent these defects and thus reduce the incidence of miscarriage. Another way in which embryo research is useful is in discovering new methods of contraception which have fewer side-effects and are more acceptable than those presently available. In view of the world's population explosion and the serious threat to human resources, this would seem to be a very desirable objective.

But these utilitarian arguments are valueless in themselves. Means are not solely justified by the ends. Opponents of this research pointed out, perfectly correctly, that utilitarian arguments of this kind – drawn to their logical conclusion – would mean that it would be acceptable to do the kind of human experimentation done by the Nazis. But if the knowledge derived from a concentration camp experiment involving the destruction of just one Jewish child was to save the lives of hundreds of other humans, the experiment would still be unacceptably evil.

So the real issue is whether the human embryo constitutes sacrosanct human life and whether this research violates it. Clearly nature herself does not regard the embryo as sacrosanct because only one in five embryos actually becomes a baby. Most fertilised eggs do not make it beyond the first menstrual period, when they are flushed out of the uterus. Certainly the embryo is human, and certainly it is alive. It also has a specific collection of genes attributable to it. However, the sperm is equally human, and unquestionably alive. Moreover it also has a unique collection of genes. One of the concerns that people have is that once fertilisation has occurred we have a unique human individual. This is what makes, it is claimed, the embryo sacred human life. But identical twinning occurs after fertilisation, and indeed can occur up to fourteen days after the egg is fertilised – long after the period of time that we can keep a human embryo in culture in the laboratory. Oddly, any one of 180 million sperm that may be simultaneously ejaculated is unique, but the embryo which comes afterwards may not be.

The Catholic Church argues that the embryo is different from egg or sperm because it is at the embryo stage when it can be claimed that it is a potential human being. Life begins at fertilisation, it maintains. I have difficulty with this because the egg also has potential,

Embryo Research and Testing for Genetic Defects

only providing it meets a sperm. The embryo has potential only providing it reaches the uterine lining. Moreover, fertilisation is not a simple instantaneous process, but in itself a continuum like the rest of existence. Is the moment of fertilisation when the sperm attaches to the egg? Is it when the egg is penetrated? Is it when the sperm head decondenses some hours later? Is it when the male and female pronucleus first appear and 18 hours after penetration. All these stages are gradual and yet the embryo still has not divided into two cells, which in itself is not a sudden process. I also find it curious that the end point of fertilisation is differently defined under British, French and German law. Certainly there is no consensus about 'when life begins'.

The Catholic position was not always so certain. St Thomas Aquinas, who died in 1274, attempted to distinguish between the flesh or substance of the embryo (Latin *caro*) and the mind or soul (Latin *anima*). He asserted that the caro was formed some time before the anima, the soul entering the body after it had been formed. It was only after ensoulment that a human had really come into existence. This is somewhat similar to the Jewish position from which Christian tradition, after all, derives. The Talmud speaks of the human embryo as 'me'a b'alma', mere fluid, up to forty days after fertilisation and suggests that a woman should not even consider herself really pregnant until then. The Jewish position seems much closer to what we as biologists actually observe, namely that the embryo and subsequently the fetus have a growing importance and status as development continues. Thus abortion is permitted to Jews under proper circumstances, for example, to save the life of a woman. Unlike the Catholic view, the fetus, right up to the moment of birth, does not have full human rights. This is practically how in British Law the embryo and subsequently the fetus are viewed if for some reason they are lost spontaneously.

There is no official mandatory mourning or burial service for a child which dies before birth. Again there is a precedent here in Jewish observance, which has extremely strict rules about what is permissible after the loss of a relative or a baby. A miscarriage, though sad, requires no fast, no statutory week of mourning, no memorial service, no sitting shiva.

So if life does not begin at fertilisation, when does it begin? My own view is that the Warnock Commission got it right. It proposed that the human embryo should be protected from the fourteenth day after fertilisation. This apparently arbitrary limit on embryo research was not nearly so capricious as has been claimed. At fourteen days, the first beginnings of organ development occur, when the primitive streak appears on the dorsal surface of the embryo. It is this structure which will eventually give rise to the embryonic nervous system. Moreover, fourteen days is when a woman would normally expect to see her period after fertilisation and is the moment when implantation can be said to have been established. It is, effectively, when pregnancy begins. Fourteen days is also more or less the last stage when twinning can occur; after this time the embryo really can be said to be individual. Finally, of course, fourteen days is the last possible time when a human embryo can live independently from its mother; after this, the placenta is needed for its nutrition and development. It would not be possible to keep a human embryo in culture beyond this stage without an artificial placenta.

The fourteen-day limit for embryo research is surely appropriate because this is the moment when we can first identify any evidence of a primitive nerve system, and thus a brain. Humanity is above all unique because of the brain. Brain activity is surely our conscience and our consciousness. This is why organs such as kidneys may be taken for donation after brain death. Once brain death has occurred, human life is regarded as finally

Embryo Research and Testing for Genetic Defects

extinguished. Perhaps the true start of human life is when brain activity begins.

There is one other argument concerning embryo research which I feel is most powerful. Some people, a minority, feel very strongly that research on the human embryo is wrong and that it debases God's creation. Others feel that the embryo has no particular status at all and that it is, for example, even perfectly acceptable to terminate pregnancy for comparatively trivial reasons well after the organs have been formed. Most people probably hold opinions between these extremes, or are not particularly concerned about these issues at all. I have genuine and deep respect for the orthodox Catholic position which regards human life as sacred. Indeed I, as an orthodox Jew, come from a similar tradition myself. The difference is that I have a different view about what constitutes human life. It is clear that biologically there can be no well-delineated definition, and Jewish tradition takes great cognizance of scientific observation when deciding relevant issues.

Had 'The Right to Life' lobby been able to force British law into banning this genetic research, it would have had a peculiar result. Most women wanting embryo screening request it because they want above all to avoid termination of pregnancy. They enter preimplantation diagnosis because they consider that if they discard a damaged embryo before implantation this is simply mimicking what generally happens in nature. Embryo screening is seen by them to be more acceptable than waiting until pregnancy is established and then having antenatal diagnosis with abortion. A Jew carrying a gene defect such as Tay-Sachs disease which affects her baby will inevitably watch that baby die of a prolonged and disgusting illness as its brain slowly deteriorates. Three years is usually the life span. But abortion of such a pregnancy would be anathema to many orthodox Jews. Not so IVF with embryo screening; this is undoubtedly acceptable under the strictest Jewish law. Indeed, the great Jewish twelfth-century philosopher Maimonides pointed out that it was our duty to prevent genetic disease if we could. Had perfectly moral fundamentalist Christians imposed their beliefs in our contemporary society, some equally moral and religious people from different traditions would have faced decisions which to them were less acceptable. In a pluralist society, we should not be too ready to impose personal moral values which may not be relevant to all caring and responsible people in that society. That is why, above all, I believe Parliament was correct with its vote in 1990.

Many opponents of embryo research suggested that our work was the beginning of a slippery slope. In 1990, it was maintained that if Parliament passed permissive legislation, within five years scientists would wish to push the frontiers back further. They would want to do experiments on more advanced embryos and would want to attempt genetic engineering. This simply has not happened. Parliamentary trust in scientists has been justified, and I believe that even without a regulatory body such as the HFEA, there would be little risk of unacceptable or unethical research being done.

An accusation which is occasionally levelled at doctors like myself is that we are practising eugenics. This is a pejorative term, which is frequently used to provoke a strong emotional reaction against our work. The term eugenics was coined by Sir Francis Galton in around 1869. The laboratory at University College, London, where ironically some our research has continued, is named after him. 'Eugenics' is derived from the Greek, meaning 'well' or 'normally' 'born'. Galton believed that it would be possible to help man's evolution and to improve the human population by 'judicious matings... to give the more suitable races or strains of blood a better chance of prevailing speedily over the less

Embryo Research and Testing for Genetic Defects

suitable.' This theory came under criticism as a form of class prejudice, but he clearly thought that by these means he could have improved the human race. Had he had a better knowledge of genetics, he might have realised that his approach was impossible and that 'selective breeding' or 'judicious matings' would not significantly improve intelligence, nor indeed any other human attribute. Galton's ideas unfortunately had a huge influence in the United States where great harm was done. In 1926, The American Eugenics Society was set up. It proposed that the wealth and social position of the upper classes was justified by superior genetic endowment. Eugenicists in the USA supported the idea that immigration from countries with 'inferior' stock such as Italy and Greece should be restricted. They called for the compulsory sterilisation of certain individuals such as 'feeble-minded', insane, epileptic and retarded American citizens. It now seems shocking that no fewer than thirty American states passed eugenic legislation, and many thousands of people were sterilised without consent, particularly in California. However bad that was, the common response to the term 'eugenics' has much to do with our reaction to the Nazis who wished to purify Germany, making it a truly Aryan nation. The Nazis were committed to the most offensive and brutal eugenic ideas, which led to their rationalising their attempts at destruction of the Jewish people with the appalling methods they devised, and their sinful treatment of gypsies, homosexuals and handicapped people. The revulsion which has been universal at their unthinkable oppression has led to the recognition that any attempt to alter our genetic heritage must be scrutinised with meticulous care.

As it happens, the eugenic approach does not work in any case. There is no serious concern that screening of embryos, no matter how widespread, would seriously change the gene pool. Galton did not understand the basic mechanism of genetics. New genetic defects occur spontaneously all the time, and even if preimplantation diagnosis was totally commonplace, it would fortunately have little effect on the population. However, it is genuinely valuable for individuals who wish to improve their chances of simply having a child that is not going to die prematurely with great suffering. Public approval for screening of this sort clearly has a very strong consensus.

Another very serious accusation that is levelled at our work is that, by screening out serious defects, we are diminishing the value and status of handicapped people. There clearly is a risk that the birth of a genetically damaged person may result in that individual being regarded as a freak. People could feel that such an individual has no right to exist, if the State sanctions attempts at a 'search and destroy' policy carried out at the start of pregnancy. Alternatively, conditions such as blindness, which are totally compatible with a rich and fulfilled life, may be seen as better to be avoided in all cases. I do not agree with this, though I agree that this is powerful argument and a criticism to which we must be sensitive. It seems to me, though, that the reasonable treatment and prevention of any disease is the concern of a doctor. That does not mean that people who are diseased or damaged in some way are less valuable to their family or to society. Fundamentally I am an optimist; I have sufficient belief in humanity to believe that it is possible to provide genetic screening when it is requested in a responsible way. This need not in any sense demean or devalue other individuals and their families who suffer the consequences of some of these diseases.

The 1990 legislation was a very important step forward. What has been achieved in the last five years? Firstly, the sexing of embryos to detect diseases which affect only one sex has been largely perfected. Remember Richard Penketh and his early attempts at staining the chromo-

Embryo Research and Testing for Genetic Defects

somes – work which Alan Handyside and I smiled at? It turns out that chromosome staining is extremely accurate and highly reliable. In fact, it is even better than PCR for chromosome disorders. In conjunction with the world-famous group at the Galton Laboratory, University College, London, led by Dr Joy Delhanty and assisted by Dr Joyce Harper, various improvements in staining techniques have been developed. We can now make a diagnosis on some chromosomal disorders within two hours. The chromosomes can be stained with brilliant fluorescent dyes and we can examine not only the sex chromosomes, but nearly all chromosome pairs. We have started successfully screening embryos for Down's syndrome (three copies of chromosome 21) and have been able to screen for some of the chromosomal defects which cause women to repeatedly miscarry. One woman who has just started this treatment has lost seven pregnancies in the last three years.

PCR has also been developed to a much more sophisticated degree. In 1991, we were lucky enough to meet Dr Mark Hughes, a clinical geneticist from Baylor College, Houston. He had been working on a number of modifications of PCR in his laboratory in Texas. He suggested a modification of PCR which would enable us, for the first time, to diagnose not merely sex, but a specific gene defect. The disease in which he was interested was cystic fibrosis. About one in twenty of the British population carry a gene for this disease. If they marry somebody with the same gene mutation, they have a risk of having an affected child. The chance of two people with mutation marrying is 1 in 20 x 20 i.e. one in 400. With a recessive disease of this kind one in four of their children will on average be affected, two out of four carriers, and one in four free of the gene mutation completely. The mathematics are simple and it means that about one in 1600 (20 x 20 x 4) children are born with cystic fibrosis. A child who is affected develops severe scarring of the lungs. Being a carrier does not matter at all, providing one is not unlucky enough to fall in love and marry somebody who by chance has the same gene.

Plans went ahead for the preimplantation diagnosis of cystic fibrosis and several couples who had lost children wrote in asking if we could help them. It soon became obvious that the slightest contamination in the PCR process was going to make diagnosis in a single cell difficult. Sometimes we could get the test to run perfectly. On other occasions we could not get it to run at all. To avoid using cells from embryos unless it was absolutely necessary, we used single white cells from carriers and affected people and single cells from the placenta. Very often the test would work perfectly in all single cells, but when we ran it in embryonic cells, it would not. It turns out that a proportion of embryonic cells have faulty DNA – this very interesting phenomenon will be discussed later in the book – and this was clearly an important limitation of the whole embryonic genetic testing process. We therefore started to test two cells taken from the embryo. Experiments were done and repeated until we were satisfied that by removing two cells from a human embryo we were not impairing its development.

By the end of 1991, we were ready to go ahead. Because we continued to have contamination problems, Mark Hughes decided that he or John Lesko, a stalwart member of his team who had never been out of the USA, would fly over from Texas bringing all their reagents, the glassware, and even bottles of absolutely clean water to ensure that the very sensitive test would work. In the event, they both came at different times to prepare everything meticulously. It was a joy to have each of them with us. Mark stayed at my house, and he immediately put up with the interminable building works that were going on, and made friends with all my

Embryo Research and Testing for Genetic Defects

children. (I think I rather impressed Mark, not because of any expertise in embryology, but because through contacts I was able to rustle up tickets for *Phantom of the Opera* at six hours' notice.) Mark comes from good Baptist stock and it was a great pleasure for all my family to see him wearing a yarmulka and joining in with the usual orthodox Jewish Friday night celebrations, welcoming the Sabbath. Dressed in cowboy kicker boots and one of my best American pullovers, looking just like a Texan, he also cooked a barbecue in my garden for the whole of the IVF team – about 80 people. It was sad about the pullover. We took him for the day to see Cambridge and to introduce him to the joys of punting. We got the punt back with Mark more or less intact, though possibly quite well lubricated, but the pullover is still probably on the bank of Clare College.

The first baby born after specific testing for any single-gene defect was from the O'Brien family, one of the first couples for whom we tried to identify the cystic fibrosis gene. The baby was born close to Manchester and rapid tests done there showed that our screening had worked. I have a very poignant photograph on my wall of this little baby at about five months old. She is smiling away. She is held in the arms of her elder brother, who looks quite ill in the photograph, suffering as he does from severe cystic fibrosis.

Many people have criticised preimplantation diagnosis on the grounds that its expense is not justified. Leaving aside any human consideration of health or happiness, this is untrue. Mark Hughes' airfare was actually paid for by United Airlines, but obviously this would not normally have been an expense. We calculate that to do the test and IVF on the O'Briens cost about £2,500. This may seem a good deal of money, but an ill child with cystic fibrosis needs special drugs, regular daily physiotherapy, antibiotics, and possibly on average three hospital admissions a year. It has been calculated that a typical child with this disease might cost the NHS around £15,000 annually. Seen in that light, our technique is certainly cost effective.

Our collaboration with Mark continued. We still felt very anxious to try to help Julie, the lady with her son strapped into a wheelchair suffering from Lesch-Nyhan syndrome. Since we had last tried to treat her, she had had two attempts at sexing embryos without success, and another termination of an affected pregnancy. As it happens, each family with Lesch-Nyhan syndrome has a slightly different configuration of the gene – the specific gene defect being a 'private mutation', that is to say that the precise DNA pattern for the defect is unique to the family. This is why we felt we would have to sex embryos, because looking for the private mutation seemed an enormously tall order. Mark was convinced that given time he could sequence the gene defect in that family. After three months hard work back in Houston, he rang me at home one night to tell me that they had cracked the sequence and were now devising a strategy involving a modification of PCR which would hopefully diagnose the defect in a single cell. After a few more weeks, they seem to have done it. Mark arranged to come to London and Julie started taking the stimulatory drugs.

The test involved running the PCR, and then after digesting the DNA with enzymes, staining the product on a piece of white blotting paper. A positive result would be pale blue; a negative result, no colour at all. Over the next week the test was repeatedly run in practice; Mark and John Lesko, who had also flown over, often worked right through the night. It soon became clear that it was going to take more than eight hours, and I was increasingly worried about keeping the embryos out of the womb that long. We were already committed to doing the biopsy on the third day, but had always managed to complete our tests so that the embryos could be transferred by 8 p.m. at the latest. We

Embryo Research and Testing for Genetic Defects

had no idea whether embryos transferred on the fourth day could implant. It was clear we would be fighting against the clock.

Julie had her egg collection and on the third day after fertilisation, five fertilised eggs were biopsied. The biopsy was difficult and one embryo disintegrated in the process. It was not until after midday that the PCR mix was ready and the DNA cookery started. At 3 p.m. we had an electrical problem – all the power in the hospital suddenly failed. It took an agonising time to have the emergency generators switched on. After further delay the PCR was restarted, but it was not until 10.45 that evening that we were ready to start the digestion, and then the staining. By 1 a.m., the stain was set up and Mark informed us that it would be another hour and a half. I decided to phone Julie to tell her to go to bed, and asked her to be at Hammersmith by 6.30 a.m. for a possible transfer. Alan, John, Mark and I retired to Alan's office which was closest to the lab. I regret to say that a certain number of cigarettes and a pipe were smoked whilst a bottle of wine and a takeaway were consumed. At around 2.15 a.m. we nervously crept into the lab. No sign of a reaction yet, so I went up to my office to return with a bottle of malt whisky. At 3 a.m. there was just the faintest shade of blue on the blotting paper – had the test worked? Mark suggested we waited another thirty minutes, and sample a bit more whisky. At 3.30 a.m., it still looked faintly blue, but then Mark pointed out that the fluorescent light might be confusing us. By 4.15 a.m., bleary-eyed, unshaven, with a headache, and feeling we might have been hallucinating, we decided to wait until there was enough natural light. By dawn it was difficult to see any trace of colour, and shortly afterwards I phoned Julie to tell her to stay in bed. The embryo was probably free of the defect, but Julie had suffered enough from appalling crises in pregnancy and I could not take such a risk.

The story does have a happy ending. A few months later, we tried again and this time things went smoothly. An apparently normal embryo was transferred. Julie now has a baby, completely healthy and free of being a carrier of the defect. This means that future generations, in this family at least, will not have to think about the appalling consequences of this disease.

Diseases like Lesch-Nyhan syndrome are devastating and completely incurable. Nor does there seem any likelihood of effective therapy in the foreseeable future. For parents the only real alternative to a very ill child, who constantly suffers and who will eventually die of the disease, has been antenatal detection and termination of pregnancy. I have no problem with termination in this kind of situation. Indeed, I believe that English law was right to recognise that different individuals may view termination with varying degrees of gravity, and to a certain extent to leave it to them to decide what is individually right. There are undoubtedly some couples, possibly not many, who with great strength and laudability would struggle to bring up a child like Peter, Julie's terribly handicapped boy. They would constantly prevent him from mutilating himself, feed him (because of course he cannot use his arms), clean him when he is incontinent, and so on. But in a family with a gene defect, a second child and a third might be conceived. Julie had actually had eight affected pregnancies.

One of the problems is, I think, that as a society we have tended to trivialise the impact of abortion. After all she had gone through, Julie felt that there was no way she could terminate another pregnancy and remain psychologically undamaged. At Hammersmith we are seeing a growing number of couples who find antenatal diagnosis unacceptable for them. Even chorion villus sampling, where testing on placental tissue can be done relatively early in pregnancy, still implies abortion after

Embryo Research and Testing for Genetic Defects

having been pregnant for three months. Amniocentesis, the removal of a fluid sample from around the baby, is generally not safe before 15–16 weeks. Diagnostic analysis of that fluid may take another three weeks, so by the time termination is to be considered, pregnancy is virtually halfway to term and the baby can be felt kicking. Moreover, both chorion villus sampling and amniocentesis involve some risk to the baby. In the last five years, I have seen seven babies miscarried by infertile women after amniocentesis. In each case, the tests were normal and the baby healthy. Of course amniocentesis may not have been responsible for the miscarriage in each case. However, the psychological effect on those parents, who did not know whether they were responsible for the destruction of their baby after years of trying to get pregnant, was very distressing to see.

This is why research continues into trying to diagnose defects at an earlier stage of pregnancy. Some scientists have tried to detect fetal cells which escape into the mother's blood stream from the placenta. Shedding of these cells can occur very early and genetic tests on those might help detection of defects. Although there has been some enthusiastic reporting in the press about this technique, there are major problems with it. Firstly, it is very difficult to separate fetal cells from the maternal blood cells, and there is a risk that the maternal DNA gives a false reading. Secondly, very few cells may get into the circulation and many of these may be dying or abnormal, giving false results. Lastly, fetal cells can apparently persist in the circulation of women who have been pregnant and it is possible that tests might simply reflect results from a pregnancy conceived before the current conception, possible as long as two or three years earlier. Other antenatal diagnostic techniques in pregnancy have been to look for cells coming away from the placenta, and thence through the cervix and into the vagina. The method of collecting fetal cells is potentially simple, not even requiring a blood test. However, most of the same problems exist, the main one being that there is a strong possibility of DNA contamination giving false results.

Consequently, there seems to be considerable merit in IVF with preimplantation diagnosis, before pregnancy begins. A woman has the great reassurance of knowing that she is getting pregnant with a healthy pregnancy. All other tests, both the ones currently done and those being researched, involve termination of pregnancy, though admittedly in some cases at quite an early stage. Undoubtedly there has been considerable demand for our technique, which is likely to grow as more women hear about it. There are now three centres in the USA doing it and one in Canada. Units in Israel, Belgium, Australia, France, Spain, and Scandinavia have started to do a few cases and it looks as if this method of screening is going to increase.

Prospective patients have at present to be cautioned very carefully about what to expect. Debbie S. is desperate to have preimplantation diagnosis, but we have to be cautious and warn her of potential pitfalls she might experience. Patients like Debbie S. have had the most harrowing time watching a baby die, and we have to be extremely careful in not overpromoting the advantages of what we are trying to do. The main concerns that any patient has to be carefully told are:

1 On average, a single treatment by IVF for preimplantation diagnosis only has a one in three chance of producing a pregnancy. Therefore, there must be recognition that the most likely outcome of any single treatment will inevitably be failure to get pregnant.
2 There may possibly be a slightly increased risk of miscarriage after preimplantation diagnosis. This is because it seems that removal of a cell from the embryo may reduce the number of cells that subsequently form to produce the placenta. This could, theoretically,

Embryo Research and Testing for Genetic Defects

make the embryo very slightly less likely to implant in the uterus properly but, at present, insufficient numbers of pregnancies have been generated to be sure about this particular risk.

3 The treatment carries a risk of twins. This is because we try, whenever possible, to transfer two embryos to give a better chance of a pregnancy. In about one-third of pregnancies, both embryos will successfully implant. Couples can, if they wish, elect to have only a single embryo transferred, but this does reduce the chance of a pregnancy.

4 The technology used for diagnosing genetic defects in embryos is almost as scientifically advanced as that on board the space shuttle! In spite of this, there cannot be any absolute guarantee that we will definitely get the diagnosis correct. We tell patients that we will only go ahead with a treatment and embryo transfer if our mathematical calculations clearly show that we have less than a 5% chance of getting things wrong. Because a small risk of having a baby which is affected by the specific defect carried in the family still remains, we advise patients to consider back-up diagnosis with amniocentesis or chorion villus sampling if they get pregnant.

5 All available research in numerous animal species clearly indicates that removal of a cell from an embryo causes no harm, and is not associated with any defects after birth. Extensive research has also been done with human embryos and we find no evidence of any serious damage. Moreover, a number of live babies have now been born and all of them have been normal, with no birth defects. In spite of all this positive evidence and in spite of getting full ethical approval for this work both locally and nationally, we still advise prospective patients that this work is experimental and that we need to be very cautious with it. For these reasons we ask patients who are undergoing this treatment to give us a commitment of allowing medical follow-up on any child born as a result of this work. We feel that this should be done on an annual basis for the time being.

As we shall see in the last chapter in this book, pre-implantation diagnosis has many important implications in the long-term. Apart from genetic screening, it is a formidable way of examining embryos to see why they do not develop properly in so many cases. There is no doubt that it will be used to investigate improvements in IVF techniques. As a genetic screening method, it is at present still in comparatively primitive stages. I am sure it will get easier and cheaper. It will become far more cost effective once we can improve IVF by growing the eggs in the laboratory from pieces of ovary, as described on page 91. It will become easier when we are able to improve the diagnostic methods of PCR. In five years both PCR and chromosome staining have improved dramatically, and there are encouraging signs that these improvements will continue and that some of the many thousands of diseases that might be prevented, will be prevented.

Chapter Five

Visions of Mortality

Joanna was happily two months pregnant when death threatened her in 1988. At her second antenatal attendance she was told that the routine pregnancy blood test she had had done contained excessive numbers of white cells. She had leukaemia, cancer of the blood. Termination of the pregnancy was discussed with her, but her doctors felt that she needed skilled advice from experts in blood diseases before taking this step. Joanna lived in Lisbon and the doctors there felt that the best expertise was in London, and my colleagues, the haematologists in the Leukaemia Unit at Hammersmith Hospital, were contacted.

Feeling sick and in a strange country, Joanna arrived at Hammersmith just eleven weeks pregnant. The pregnancy was doing fine. Joanna's general condition was excellent and the leukaemia team felt that they could manage for the time being with drugs and by washing her blood. Over the next five months Joanna literally commuted between Lisbon and London for repeated treatment and for antenatal care. In August 1988, we did a Caesarean section and Veronica, a lovely dark-haired girl of 7 lb 10 oz (3.275 kg), was delivered. Joanna was started on anti-leukaemia drugs and returned temporarily to Portugal with her baby.

Joanna was incredibly lucky. As well as a brief respite from the leukaemia, and a healthy baby girl, our haematologists had found that Joanna's sister had the same tissue type. This meant she could be the ideal bone marrow donor, offering Joanna the possibility of a real cure of the disease. One problem about a bone marrow transplant was, though, that she would need a carefully administered but massive dose of irradiation to her entire body first. This risky manoeuvre would be needed to kill all the leukaemia cells she was producing. It would also have serious side-effects. Joanna was able to cope with the idea of these side-effects and the risk of death if the radiation went wrong. However, in common with many other young people in a similar situation she was extremely distressed at the thought that the irradiation would sterilise her. She was only twenty-three years old and this would make her menopausal.

Joanna desperately wanted Veronica to have a brother or sister. She asked if it would be possible to delay the bone marrow transplant for a while and continue with drugs in the hope that she might conceive again. Our haematologists, though concerned, agreed and in January 1989 she became pregnant again. At the beginning of March she had a miscarriage, and the doctors in Lisbon scraped out her uterus. She continued to bleed heavily and repeatedly fainted. Blood tests showed that the leukaemia was getting worse, and by mid-March she was back in London. By now time was running out, and the haematologists asked my team if we would be prepared to collect some eggs from Joanna, fertilise them with her husband's sperm and freeze the embryos for later transfer, if Joanna was cured of her disease.

Such a manoeuvre had never been done successfully before anywhere in the world. I saw Joanna and explained my general reservations about embryo freezing, described on page 28 of this book. I warned her that each frozen embryo only had around a 2% chance of being a baby, even in somebody who would not have had irradiation of this magnitude. I also felt it probable that irradiation might damage her uterus and make success even less likely. There was no definite evidence of this as early as 1989 but, as events later turned out, I was right to be so pessimistic. I explained to Joanna what the then legal status of her embryos would be, and gently explored what she would want doing with them if she did not survive. Joanna was typically brave and focused;

she temporarily stopped the anti-leukaemia drugs, started fertility injections to stimulate her ovaries and underwent an IVF cycle.

At this stage we were lucky. In spite of the leukaemia, and all the drugs that Joanna had taken to kill leukaemia cells, the ovaries responded brilliantly and we collected no fewer than twenty-four eggs. Of these, thirteen fertilised normally. The laboratory procedures were carefully supervised by Karin Dawson, our principal embryologist and laboratory manager, and Kevin Lindsay, the scientist in charge of our sperm lab. Karin worked most of the night to freeze all thirteen embryos in the hope that at least one or two would survive if they were subsequently thawed. Karin is a remarkable and dedicated manager – she is really the secret weapon at Hammersmith which gives our laboratories such an edge. She is quite bossy but incredibly caring – everybody on the unit calls her 'mother' – I think of her as Kanga, the A.A. Milne character. The embryos were placed in long-term storage in liquid nitrogen, and Joanna was ready to restart anti-leukaemic drugs.

I will not go into the details of the total body radiation therapy that Joanna had later that year. Suffice it to say that she was, of course, extremely sick. She suffered a good deal of chest and abdominal pain. She lost her voice and, of course, had the usual problems with hair loss and severely itchy skin rashes. The good news was that her bone marrow transfusion from her sister appeared to take, and she was starting to produce new blood cells free of leukaemia. Her recovery was gradual, though, and she continued to feel nauseated and have no appetite for many weeks; she also had continual shaking of her body and her hands. One thing that worried the haematologists was that her skin rash persisted and was still severe two months after the transplant. What was happening was that she had developed graft versus host disease – a possibly fatal complication. Now that Joanna had lost all her own white blood cells, she had no immunity of her own. Her immunity was from her sister's white cells and these cells were actually rejecting Joanna's own tissues.

Massive drug treatment with steroids was started and this did the trick. Joanna remained very tired and sick, but her diarrhoea improved as did the skin rash. Eighteen weeks after the bone marrow transplant, though not fully well, she was able to return to Lisbon, agreeing to return to London at very frequent intervals for regular supervision. Within one year her strength was largely recovered. Her weight was close to what it had been before radiotherapy and, apart from mouth ulcers, she was fit, with no evidence of leukaemia and no apparent rejection. She felt well enough even tentatively to raise the possibility of another pregnancy with the doctors.

By January 1992, Joanna was feeling pretty good. She had stopped all her drugs except antibiotics, as she had little natural resistance against infection. It was now well over two years since her leukaemia treatment and there was no sign of recurrence. She booked an appointment with us for March to have an attempt at embryo transfer. By now, of course, she was menopausal, and her uterus was inactive. We started her on the hormone replacement therapy needed to make her uterus receptive to the embryos. Over the next few weeks, the ultrasound confirmed my original fears. In spite of large doses of oestrogen, her uterus would not respond and the womb lining was not growing sufficiently thick to allow an embryo to implant and support a pregnancy. Repeated measurements showed that the lining was no more than 4 millimetres thick – the normal being above 11 milli-metres. Clearly the radiation damage was severe and almost certainly irreversible. We cancelled the transfer.

She returned two months later and we tried to stimulate her uterus again. After fourteen days of much heavier hormone therapy, there was still no response from the uterine lining and certainly every indication that an embryo transfer would fail. We cancelled the transfer and arranged to try the following month, in July. We restimulated her and she continuously had more than a double dose of oestrogen. Blood tests revealed that the oestrogen levels in her blood stream were very high and that the oestrogen must be therefore getting to the right place. Once again, though, the uterus had failed to respond and its thickness was 5 millimetres. Rather than waste the precious embryos by a seemingly futile transfer, we abandoned the thawing procedure for the third time. My close friend and colleague Mr Margara decided to give her a quick anaesthetic and scrape the uterus.We hoped that examining tissue from the lining would tell us whether or not it was developing at all normally. Very little lining was recovered at the scrape. Microscopic examination of the tissue revealed very inactive endometrium with a poor hormonal response. I told Joanna that I felt very gloomy about any prospect of pregnancy. I suggested that she should continue to take hormone replacement therapy for at least six months, in the rather forlorn hope that her uterus might recover a bit. I made no secret of my pessimism, but privately was even more certain there was no chance of success.

Joanna returned in May 1993. She had been on regular hormone therapy. We immediately increased the dose she was given until her blood levels of oestrogen reached extraordinary heights – indeed, I have never had a patient with such levels. I was amazed she felt so well. We also discussed the idea of giving her other hormones, as well including more progesterone in her hormone 'diet'. Regular daily ultrasound was started. It was now well into June and still the uterine lining remained implacably at between four and five millimetres only, far too thin normally for pregnancy. At this point Joanna begged me to transfer her embryos, whatever the situation. She felt that she could not continue in limbo any longer. I remembered from animal research that sometimes embryos could implant in a highly inapprop-riate tissue; I also knew that human embryos could occasionally implant where there was no endometrium at all, for example, in the tube where ectopic pregnancy occurs. I agreed to try an embryo transfer because there seemed no alternative. Immediately, Joanna asked that all her embryos be thawed. We pointed out to her that they could not be frozen a second time and that we could only transfer two, or at most three, into her uterus. She was adamant; she felt that she wanted to give things one last go, and that if this did not work, she said, she would return to Portugal and look after her only child, Veronica.

A final large dose of hormones was given. Joanna was asked to stand by, ready for her transfer, and Karin prepared the lab before finally taking the embryos out of their liquid nitrogen container, where they had been for the last four years. Karin tells me that at this stage she felt extremely reluctant to do things this way; she really had difficulty accepting that it was Joanna's specific wish that all the embryos should be thawed. She kept on thinking of the waste this involved, but felt obliged to comply with Joanna's request. The first embryo was removed and slowly thawed. In disbelief, Karin watched it disintegrate under the microscope. The second embryo was taken out, and the same thing happened. With growing distress, Karin watched the third, then the fourth embryo break up as they were thawed. It was now clear that Joanna had come all this way, had survived all this treatment, and that we were likely to have nothing to return to her damaged uterus.

By the time the seventh embryo was being thawed, Karin was in despair, wondering how she was going to tell Joanna that all this treatment, all this hope, had been completely illusory. But under the microscope, this embryo seemed as if it might be viable. She quickly processed the medium in which it needed to be cultured and placed in the incubator. Of the remaining six embryos, no fewer than three looked as if they could possibly have survived. These three, together with the other apparently viable embryo, were left overnight in the incubator.

The following day, the embryos were inspected. Each had divided perfectly and, remarkably, seemed to be growing absolutely normally. Joanna was telephoned and she came up to the hospital. Her uterine lining was no better on ultrasound, but we were now committed to doing the transfer. The three best embryos were chosen for return to her uterus. This was an obvious decision – whilst normally we would have transferred only two, the chance of a pregnancy was obviously so remote that we clearly had to transfer the maximum number the law permitted. The fourth was left in culture, where after a few days it naturally disintegrated. Joanna was given a special booster hormone injection and after an hour resting in the unit on a couch returned to where she was staying in London.

Joanna remained in London, giving us a blood sample on the fifteenth day after the embryo transfer. Late that same afternoon, Dinah, our hormone assay technician, ran into my office shouting in her usual excitable way. Joanna's blood test suggested pregnancy; moreover, the hormone level was so high that it seemed that it could actually be that two embryos had implanted. It is difficult to describe the telephone conversation with Joanna and her husband that evening. I repeatedly advised her to be very cautious, because I felt sure that a miscarriage was probable, but her elation was not controllable. Within a few days we repeated the blood tests (they were strongly positive) and then, two weeks later an ultrasound confirmed that two babies were indeed growing; Joanna had twins. Again, we all repeatedly advised extreme caution, none of us, of course, wanting to see these remarkable hopes dashed. We all agreed that it would be in Joanna's best interests if she remained in London for the time being, and Joanna made arrangements for Veronica to have continued care by other family members in Lisbon.

Three weeks passed before disaster struck. Joanna started to bleed vaginally. A scan taken rapidly showed that the first twin was not thriving, and it looked as if a miscarriage was about to happen. I filled Joanna full of a drug which I hoped might encourage the babies to stay implanted. A few days later, and the first baby's heart finally stopped beating. Shortly afterwards, her bleeding also stopped and the remaining baby seemed to be surviving. Eight more weeks into pregnancy, and by now, Joanna was gaining weight. By sixteen weeks of pregnancy things looked stable, and we felt that Joanna could return to see Veronica in Lisbon, who by this time was missing her mother desperately. We had a tricky decision to make, but finally I felt that this baby really had to be delivered in London. The pregnancy was still high risk, and both Joanna and her husband were grateful that we felt that we should arrange to deliver her here. The plan was for her to get antenatal care with a very good doctor I knew in Lisbon, and for her to return at about 32 weeks of pregnancy – some two months before the baby was due.

I was away at an international meeting when Joanna returned to London in January 1994. She was fit and well and the pregnancy was coming along nicely. As I nowadays do almost no pregnancy care and seldom deliver a baby myself, she was booked to see my new senior registrar, who did the usual checks. The haematologists also examined her and found that from their point of view she was entirely fit. Arrangements were made for her to have routine weekly antenatal visits in the out-patients at Hammersmith. It was now that I had an incredible piece of luck. The following Tuesday, I was most unusually free. Two new patients had failed to keep their appointments and, completely uncharacteristically and to prevent myself from jumping up and down in frustration at the waste of time, I found myself wandering through the out-patient waiting room chatting to one or two couples. Suddenly, I saw Joanna, who I had forgotten was back in London, waiting patiently for her antenatal appointment with my registrar. She was sitting in a far corner of the waiting room and, to me, who by now knew her well, she looked very off colour. Her face was unusually puffy and she looked really quite bloated. She said she felt absolutely fine. I asked her if she would help me kill time and showed her into my consulting room. A quick check of her blood pressure showed that it was a bit raised, but the pregnancy seemed well enough. Alarm bells about her odd appearance started to ring in my head, but I kept on thinking I was being ridiculously neurotic. I asked her whether she might be prepared to come into hospital for a few tests. She seemed perfectly happy with the idea and asked what time tomorrow. Feeling even more foolish, and really without good clinical reason, I suggested she came in straight away and that she sent for her night clothing. I rang the antenatal ward to say I was admitting a patient, handed Joanna her notes and suggested she went straight upstairs, accompanied by a nurse from the clinic.

By the time Joanna got to the ward and into bed, fifteen minutes later, her blood pressure was sky high. A urine test by the nurse revealed a huge amount of protein in the urine. Joanna had a rare condition called fulminating pre-eclampsia. This is very serious for the baby because its blood supply is seriously threatened, and such babies frequently die. Severe toxaemia of this sort can also be fatal for the mother, or result in a stroke because of the sudden blood pressure increase. We do not understand the cause of this very severe form of toxaemia of pregnancy, which usually only occurs in a first pregnancy. It is thought to be related to the response of the immune system and is very rare in a second pregnancy unless the woman is having a child by a new partner. In Joanna's case she had already had Veronica, but we knew for certain that this was her husband's child because we had fertilised the eggs four years earlier. However, since the irradiation and transplant, Joanna's immune system was no longer her own. She had the white cells produced by her sister's bone marrow. This was the only logical explanation for this extreme emergency.

Over the next few hours, Joanna's kidneys started to fail and she retained fluid. Her face became so puffy that she was hardly recognisable. We had sedated her heavily and, with drugs, had brought her blood pressure under relative control. I was now faced with a difficult, but really inevitable, decision. It was clear that Joanna's life was at serious risk. Moreover, this small premature baby could die at any moment. Given that her blood pressure had temporarily settled – and before it veered out of control again – I would need to do an emergency Caesarean section. But this one remaining baby was only at thirty-three weeks. Clearly there was a risk that it might not survive; for that, we were going to have to rely on the excellent paediatric team at Hammersmith, who are so skilled with very small babies.

On 18 January 1994, Matilda, weighing just over 4 lb (1.75 kilograms), was born. She was the first baby born in the world after cancer treatment with irradiation of the mother and embryo freezing. Within an hour of birth she did not even need an incubator, or any special oxygen supply. Joanna immediately started to recover. Her kidneys began to make urine, though it was to be nearly two weeks before her blood pressure reached safe limits. I am a Jew, so I am moderately used to warm family gatherings to welcome the new infant, with various relatives clucking over the baby and fussing over the mother. I was not, however, prepared for the Portuguese family which had gathered in Joanna's room when I walked into it the following day. There was her mother and father, as well as her husband's parents, and delightful little Veronica in little pigtails. All had flown over from Lisbon and, though anxious about Joanna, who was still very swollen with fluid, they showed me just how much they cared about what had happened to Joanna and how grateful they were to the Hammersmith's nurses and doctors.

My favourite pastime is skiing, and I go to the Alps whenever I can. Generally, ten of us from the team go together in the winter, and usually I take one of my children with us – part of my real family and my extended family together. On this occasion, the haematologists stole a trick on me. Within a month of Matilda's birth, the haematology team sent me an abstract of a paper they were going to present at a big leukaemia meeting in Davos. Lectures about blood diseases were not the only activity that was intended. My name was on the paper as a co-author, but none of the haematologists was suggesting that my presence was in any way essential for their presentation. I just prayed that they would have no snow.

Joanna's story has not ended. She returned to Lisbon with her family in February, buoyant and hopeful. In April 1994, I was in my office when, looking through the open door, I saw Joanna sobbing outside. She had come back for a routine check-up in the leukaemia clinic. Although she felt totally well in herself, tests had confirmed that there were some new leukaemia cells in her blood. Obviously another major treatment of the sort she had already had was not going to be possible but, she told me, the haematologists planned a new treatment. There was hope that her blood might respond to transfusions of her sister's white cells. Over this last year, this has been done repeatedly, and things seem to be under control. I last saw Joanna four months ago when she seemed quite well. Her last letter to me was subdued but hopeful, but nobody can predict what the future holds for her.

I have told Joanna's story in unusual detail. Firstly, I want to pay tribute to an incredibly brave woman and a wonderful mother. Secondly, she exemplifies what some people are prepared to go through to have a baby. Lastly, I feel that her story sharply focuses many of the problems which these new reproductive techniques bring.

As cancer treatments become more successful, there is a growing awareness that, in both young men and women, one of the main complications is the inevitable sterility caused by radiation therapy, and occasionally by the drug treatment (chemotherapy) which kills the cancer cells. What is at first rather surprising is that for many young women the thought of possible sterility is much more distressing than the thought that their cancer may kill them. In Joanna's case, she was fully prepared to delay life-saving treatment to go through an egg collection and have her embryos frozen. This to her was more acceptable than considering the possibility of a donated egg from another individual later in life. We see the same thing in the case of Rebecca, another incredibly brave young woman. She developed cancer of the lymph glands whilst still a student, and it was clear from the very beginning that her form of tumour was extremely aggressive and rapidly spreading. Throughout the time when she was dealing with the idea that she might well die before her twentieth birthday, she was consumed with the notion that she must protect her fertility at all costs. Her treatment started before she had a husband, and therefore embryo freezing was not an option. When she had her initial illness in 1985, both egg freezing and freezing of pieces of ovary had not even been considered experimentally. For her, the only option was a major abdominal operation to move her ovaries upwards out of her pelvis, so that when her lymph glands were irradiated, the ovaries would be outside the beam of radiation. I did this operation quite experimentally; an operation that Rebecca knew had not really been previously tried for her kind of serious illness. Throughout, her main concern was whether the operation had worked, rather than the thought that the radiation might not save her life. In fact, in the next five years, Rebecca had four recurrences of her cancer and each time needed massive therapy. On each occasion, the thing that she found most distressing was the thought that she would never have a child. These feelings of Rebecca's – so similar to those experienced by Joanna – seem to argue that failure to conceive in such circumstances is a kind of final confirmation of a person's complete mortality.

Such feelings bring strong pressures on doctors. There is, quite reasonably, major pressure from cancer patients to freeze sperm, eggs or embryos as a hedge against future infertility. In our laboratories at Hammersmith we have a huge number of sperm samples, stored in liquid nitrogen, given by men who are about to undergo radiation or chemotherapy. At the time when these samples are preserved it may be difficult, or indeed impossible, to have detailed discussions with the patient concerning all the implications of what he is about to do. Firstly, the act of preservation may be a last-minute decision, taken at a time when all sorts of conflicting emotions are rapidly maturing. Secondly, it may not be sensible or kind to spell out to such distressed patients what should be done with their sperm or embryos in the event of their death due to failure of the cancer treatment.

I think this is one of the considerations that persuaded Joanna to suddenly insist that all her embryos were thawed, come what may. Having faced her possible mortality for some time, she was suddenly able to come to a very mature decision. I do not think she wanted her husband to have the problem of deciding what to do about her unique and precious embryos in the event of her death from leukaemia. If she got pregnant, well and good. If she did not, a potential problem she was bequeathing to her family would be simply solved.

Let me end this chapter with another example of this problem, a type of problem I see with increasing frequency. Although the story does not concern an actual cancer sufferer, I think it illustrates the problems that are raised very well. Marilyn was happily married to Jonathan when he developed a rare but fatal genetic disease. It happens that this genetic disease is a disorder which is passed on to 50% of a sufferer's children. The children are either entirely healthy, or they die of the illness. The gene cannot yet be detected so antenatal or embryonic diagnosis is not yet possible. Unusually for a genetic disorder, the disease from which Jonathan suffered does not normally manifest itself in childhood, but in early adulthood, and after a horrific lingering illness – which can last a few years – they invariably die. I shall not describe this disease – for one thing its effects are fairly disgusting. For another, because it is so rare, it might enable a knowledgeable reader to identify the family concerned which would be an invasion of their privacy.

In the throes of his last illness and in the hope that a particular experimental treatment might work, Jonathan gave sperm for freezing knowing that the treatment would undoubtedly make him sterile. This sperm subsequently found its way to my laboratories because we had long-term storage facilities. The physicians looking after him certainly encouraged him to donate sperm for storage and, under the circumstances, who can blame them. As far as I am aware, consideration of what to do with his sperm if he died was not fully discussed with him or with his wife. Nor, I believe, was there much discussion about the 50:50 chance of any child getting the same illness when he or she grew up.

The experimental treatment failed and Jonathan died. Marilyn loved him dearly and continued to grieve. One year after his death, Jonathan's doctors sent her to me because she was repeatedly asking to have insemination with her dead husband's sperm. Jonathan's doctors had suddenly got cold feet as they realised the implications – namely that there was a 50% chance that any child born might carry the gene. They were hoping that I would talk her out of this decision, as I would be the person in charge of the insemination.

When Marilyn came to see me I was struck by her personality and also by her beauty. From the start it was clear that she was going to demand the insemination, whatever I advised. I suggested that it might be premature to go for her husband's child so soon after his death, and suggested that at the very least she waited to make sure that was what she wanted. She refused all suggestions of going to seek a counsellor's help, and agreed to see me in six months. After two further visits and a year had elapsed, I was more and more convinced I could not morally justify much further delay in my decision. Marilyn said that, firstly, this was what she and her husband had privately agreed. Secondly, she said, there was no possibility of her wanting to find another husband. Thirdly, she said that although there was no treatment for this disease at present, if her child was unlucky enough to be affected, there might be a cure found in ten or fifteen years' time. Finally, she maintained that, irrespective of any legal position, the semen was effectively her responsibility as Jonathan's next-of-kin. Whilst talking to her, I was more and more convinced that to her her husband was effectively alive in the liquid nitrogen in my laboratory and that until the sperm either produced a pregnancy or was destroyed, Marilyn would remain in limbo. There could practically be no resolution for Marilyn until something definitive was done.

Just at this time, I received a letter from the consultant who had treated Marilyn:

Dear Professor Winston,
As the physician responsible for the genetic counselling of several members of this family, I have received pleas from several members of the family that any procedure using Jonathan's sperm should not be performed. The family are planning to make a formal written complaint.

Whereas I am not concerned here about the issue of whether a widowed woman should have the right to use the sperm of her dead husband, the problem is the 50% risk of any child inheriting a fatal genetic disease. I am deeply anxious for the future health and happiness of Marilyn, her prospective child, and the rest of Jonathan's family...

Finally, I am concerned about the sort of adverse publicity a case such as this might bring to my hospital as well as your own, in the present social and political climate... I hope you will give some consideration to these various issues which seem important to me in view of my knowledge of this disease and of its behaviour and effects in this family.
Yours sincerely
Dr John Able

I make no particular judgment about this letter. However, it does occur to me that the physician concerned might have considered much more carefully before referring Jonathan for sperm preservation. His 'deep anxiety for the health and happiness of Marilyn' seems to me to be coming rather late. This letter seems to me to highlight so many of the problems raised by all the advances in human reproduction, and also some of the attitudes from which certain members of my profession have not yet managed to escape.

Firstly, what right do extended family members have over the sperm or eggs of their relative? Surely very little, and if any person has the right to decide it must above all be the spouse – in this case Marilyn. In spite of the sentiments in this letter, it seems outrageous that an extended family should be able to decide or dictate against the wishes of the next of kin of the deceased person. In this case, Marilyn had lost the most, had the strongest need to grieve, and was almost certainly the only person with whom Johnathan had discussed the fate of his spermatozoa and the possibility of his offspring being raised after his death.

Secondly, how far should our respect for a patient's wishes be taken? Marilyn was adamantly prepared to allow her child to have a 50% chance of a terrible disease. What is our responsibility in this situation – to what extent do considerations for the welfare of any child, not yet born and not yet a patient, overrule our respect for the autonomy of our patient? I have dealt with this issue elsewhere in this book, but it occurs to me that it may possibly have been better to have existed in reasonable health for a while than never to have existed at all.

Thirdly, what regard should doctors have for public opinion and the reputation of a hospital, and should this act over and above their concern for the best welfare of the individual patient? I think that Dr Able, in the last paragraph of his letter, was reduced to offering a form of blackmail. Not to achieve the best welfare of the patient in the face of public opinion is to do the patient harm. To do the patient harm in such circumstances, and in the face of such pressures, is contrary to the whole ethos of my profession and, in my opinion, inadmissible.

Perhaps the real message is that before preserving eggs or sperm or embryos for anybody, and particularly from a patient suffering a potentially fatal illness, we need to take very careful stock indeed. We need to consider the implications of life suspended in the deepfreeze.

You may like to know what decision I took in Marilyn's case. I confess to my shame that I ducked the issue. My team were equally anxious about the implications of this treatment, and I decided on a compromise. I told Marilyn that I could not contemplate undertaking a major procedure like in vitro fertilisation to get her pregnant with her husband's sperm. I told her that I had real misgivings about such action. I did say, however, that I would be prepared to undertake insemination with the thawed sperm. I warned, however, that the chances of a pregnancy were low because the sperm had been taken when Jonathan was already quite ill and when he had had much drug therapy. In the event, we prepared for insemination and thawed the sperm. It was of extremely poor quality and not much in amount.

Marilyn did not get pregnant. I hope she has found resolution and that by using up all the sperm, she has finally come to terms with her husband's death. Perhaps only now is he truly buried. For my part, I still feel inadequate. I feel guilty at not being able to commit myself to a more definite decision – even though it almost certainly could have made no difference in the long run.

Freezing technology is extremely powerful and very frequently used. In fact, most IVF clinics freeze some sperm or embryos. In some cases it can provide a remarkable result, as in the case of Joanna's family. Even if something bad now happened to Joanna, I am convinced that the birth of Matilda was absolutely right, and that she will be well looked after. In Rebecca's case, had egg freezing been available, it probably would have been a real boon. But in Jonathan's case, I think this powerful technology overtook my profession's ability to foresee the fruit of our actions, and the results were painful, almost disastrous. Perhaps foreseeing the fruits of one's actions is what much of this treatment is about.

Chapter Six

IVF in Older Women

As we age we become less fertile. In men this process is gradual; many men in their seventies are very fertile, and there are recorded instances of men over ninety having fathered a child. Generally, though, as a man gets older, the manufacture of new sperm by the testicle becomes less efficient and more and more of his sperm have chromosomal abnormalities. These often prevent them from being capable of normal fertilisation. In women the whole process is much more acute. The oldest woman in Britain ever to have a baby after natural conception was fifty-four years old. Unlike men, who continue to make new sperm throughout reproductive life, the female is born with her complete complement of eggs already formed in the ovaries. These eggs are in a quiescent state of development, and their final stage of maturation starts about six months before ovulation. The great majority of the eggs in the ovary are never ovulated. They simply degenerate and are not used, a process of aging starting from birth. A baby girl begins life with about four or five million eggs in her ovaries; by puberty she only has some 400,000 left although she will not yet have ovulated once. Over the next thirty years, these remaining eggs will gradually disappear, whether ovulated or not. Finally, by the time of the menopause, no viable eggs are left in the ovaries.

The key time is the ten to fifteen years before the menopause, which usually occurs in British women around fifty years old. It is then that a woman becomes progressively less fertile. There are a number of reasons for this, but perhaps the most important is to do with a diminishing supply of good fertile eggs in the ovary. As a woman ages, she appears to ovulate eggs which are less able to be fertilised and if they are fertilised, more likely to be defective. This is why miscarriage is much more common when older women get pregnant; the embryo is more likely to have defects which result in failure of development. Similarly, this is why older women are more prone to having children which have a chromosomal abnormality. In most cases chromosomal abnormalities are not compatible with life and a pregnancy does not continue. However, trisomy 21 (three copies of chromosome 21) which causes Down's syndrome (see Chapter 4) is not incompatible with life and many of these fetuses survive to become babies, with the characteristic defects associated with this disease. A woman at thirty-five years old has about a one in 200 chance of a pregnancy with Down's syndrome. By the age of forty this risk has risen to about one in eighty and by age forty-five to about one in thirty.

As far as we know, abnormal eggs are the main reason why older women find it difficult to get pregnant. However, there are a few other important contributory reasons. Ovulation itself occurs less often because of subtle hormonal changes and the menstrual periods often become irregular. Consequently, even when an embryo is formed, the lining of the uterus may not have been adequately prepared for implantation to occur. The uterus of older women is also more likely to be abnormal. About one-third of all women have benign tumours, called fibroids, in their uterus by the time they are forty. These swellings seldom cause symptoms or serious problems but they often distort the uterus or make its blood supply rather abnormal. This is thought to increase the likelihood of infertility. Another uterine disease is adenomyosis. This scarring disorder which often causes heavy and sometimes painful periods is a benign uterine disease most commonly occurring in women between thirty-five and forty-five. It is frequently associated with infertility and is thought to interfere with the way the embryo grows or implants.

IVF in Older Women

Older women also tend to be less fertile because they are rather more likely to have sex less frequently. As we get older, we nearly all of us tend to get slightly less interested in sex, and there is no doubt that decreased sexual activity is a fairly frequent cause of infertility. Regular, frequent sex is probably of key importance in older women who want to conceive. This is because ovulation is less regular and its timing unpredictable; conception will therefore be more likely if sperms are more frequently present in the cervical mucus and uterine and tubal fluids.

The best infertility treatment for most older women is unquestionably IVF. IVF was, of course, mainly developed as a treatment to bypass damaged fallopian tubes. However, it is also the safest way to improve egg production and in older women there are fewer eggs which would be capable of giving a viable embryo. By stimulating the ovaries vigorously, several eggs can normally be produced, and the embryologist has the chance of choosing the embryos which are most likely to be able to implant. Simply stimulating the ovaries without IVF (for example, by giving fertility drugs) is not helpful and can be dangerous in this situation. This is because it does not give an opportunity to pick out the few healthy eggs that may be produced, and because the use of fertility drugs alone in sufficient doses to increase fertility in a woman who is already ovulating creates a serious risk of triplets or quadruplets – a potentially dangerous complication in an older woman.

Unfortunately, although IVF is the best treatment for older women, it is also much less likely to be successful than it is in a younger patient. Older women produce fewer eggs even with heavy stimulation, and some cannot be stimulated successfully at all. Older women also tend to produce embryos which are less likely to be viable and continue to grow to the fetal stage. Some clinics try to get around these problems by offering donated eggs to older women, but egg donors are in very short supply. Another problem is that, with or without donor eggs, IVF does not treat any underlying uterine abnormality. After fertilisation, embryos may be transferred to an environment which will not easily support their survival. Miscarriage is very much more likely after successful IVF, though the risks of miscarriage are reduced if the eggs are donated by a younger woman. The recent figures from the HFEA (1994 report) show the generally disappointing results of IVF in older women when donor eggs were not used:

	Cycles treated	Pregnant %	Live birth %	Miscarried %
Under 25	178	16.9	9.6	43
25–29	2416	22.1	16.5	25
30–34	6806	19.0	14.6	23
35–39	6039	15.2	11.4	25
40–44	2065	8.2	4.5	45
Over 45	174	3.4	1.7	50

When donor eggs were used:

	Cycles treated	Pregnant %	Live birth %	Miscarried %
Under 25	8	37.5	37.5	0
25–29	55	16.4	7.3	25
30–34	134	27.6	20.9	24
35–39	128	25.8	24.2	6
40–44	142	16.9	12.7	25
Over 45	79	25.3	17.7	30

In older women (and curiously in very much younger ones as well) the risk of miscarriage is close to double the normal risk after an IVF treatment.

The risk of being infertile due simply to aging does not seem to have frightened many women into trying to start a family sooner. In the 1950s and 60s, women throughout Western Europe tended to have their first child in their twenties. Nowadays, in most European countries including Britain, women often leave trying to have their children until later on in reproductive life. A background factor clearly is the widespread availability of relatively efficient contraception. People are having fewer children and are able, if they wish, to space out their pregnancies. There are a number of reasons for this, possibly the most significant being the growing number of women in employment, or seeking a career. Men and women are tending to form permanent relationships later in life and the age at marriage is also increasing. For all these reasons, pregnancy is frequently being deferred until a woman is in her late thirties or forties.

All this has had a powerful impact on infertility medicine. When I first started at Hammersmith twenty-five years ago, it was rare to see a woman over forty in the infertility clinic, and even rarer to offer treatment. It was usually regarded as a pointless exercise, because of the very much reduced fertility that older women have. My old boss at Hammersmith, Professor John McClure Browne, who was a terrifying and austere figure on superficial acquaintance, but extraordinarily kind and understanding with staff and patients under the distant exterior, was unusual in offering treatment to older patients quite frequently. Privately we used to say that it was because he was old himself. That his attitude was very unusual at the time is clear from the fact that most of his colleagues referred to his treatment as 'futility treatment', rather than 'fertility treatment'. Following Professor Browne's example, we did do the occasional operation to unblock tubes in forty-year-olds, but this was usually in a forlorn (and probably misguided) attempt to offer a woman some peace of mind rather than because we thought she would get pregnant. Things are very different today. Now over 25% of the female patients I see are over forty. Most of them have delayed having children; many have comparatively

Anna and Jack

Anna is a theatre director who followed her successful career in the theatre as a director until late into child-bearing life. She was forty-one at the time of her first attendance at our clinic and her experience is in many ways typical of many women having infertility treatment later in life.

She had been fully investigated for infertility at another hospital, before being referred to Hammersmith for IVF. Her partner Jack had already had a child and his sperm proved to be in excellent condition in tests. Telescope inspection of Anna's fallopian tubes had revealed earlier that her tubes were incompletely blocked. Tubal surgery was considered, but it was agreed by her doctors that the tubes were too badly damaged for surgery to have much chance of success. Many years ago she had had a coil inserted into her uterus and it is likely that this led to the infection which resulted in the infertility. An irony of her situation is that in the distant 1960s, Anna campaigned for contraception and abortion on demand.

By the time we were able to do IVF, Anna was already forty-two, at an age when the chance of success is much reduced because of the quality of the eggs in the ovaries. Her first IVF treatment went fairly well, when eleven eggs were collected and seven fertilised. Two of these looked reasonably good and were growing apparently normally. Anna and Jack elected to have them transferred, but although there was a slight rise of pregnancy hormone on the twelfth day after transfer, she sadly had a very early miscarriage. In spite of the severe disappointment, Anna found IVF a comparatively positive experience and was only too ready to try again. Four months later a second cycle was attempted.

At the second IVF attempt, thirteen eggs were collected and eleven fertilised. Ten of the embryos had grown comparatively well, which is unusual when eggs are collected from women in their forties – such a large number of potentially viable embryos being comparatively rare. It was clear that transfer of more than two embryos together was unjustified – the risk of triplets would be high, increasing the physical risk of pregnancy, particularly in a woman over forty. Because of her age, it was obvious to my team that Anna could not go through IVF repeatedly, and on the day of transfer they sought permission to freeze her remaining embryos. This was regarded as an insurance policy in case she did not become pregnant with the two 'fresh' embryos. Anna and Jack, forced to take something of a snap decision, decided to allow the spare embryos to be frozen.

Happily, Anna conceived and both embryos implanted. However, as commonly happens in older women, one of the twin implants stopped growing very soon after implantation and Anna had a term pregnancy, her baby Nina being born by Caesarean section. Even though the birth of her baby brought great fulfilment to Anna, she continued to have serious anxieties about the embryos that we had frozen and felt that she had been railroaded into a decision at the most stressful time of her treatment – the embryo transfer. It is quite clear that, with hindsight, this was something we should have discussed in much more detail with her before the treatment was under way.

recently found themselves in their 'life partnership'. These women present us with a very significant problem because they are much harder to treat. In many cases, their basic fertility by this age is now so low that no treatment, including IVF, is likely to work. There is a cruel paradox here. They may well by now be in a much better financial position to afford private treatment, but their physical position makes success much less likely.

One of the problems is, undoubtedly, that their expectations have been raised. The publicity given to IVF, and the general and public optimism surrounding all forms of fertility treatment, has led these women into believing that getting pregnant is now much easier. Every week yet another newspaper proclaims successful IVF in a slightly aging actress or film-star, or twins born to a woman close to the menopause.

But the most damaging publicity has been that given to the treatment of women well past the natural menopause. Nothing has stirred public comment so much as the issue of infertility treatment for these much older women. Remarkably, it would now be possible to get a seventy-year-old woman pregnant. When it was announced in the newspapers that Dr Antinori in Italy had now 'successfully treated a sixty-three-year-old woman', this was heralded as a great breakthrough of scientific importance. It was almost as if Dr Antinori had pioneered some remarkable new treatment. It was, of course, nothing of the kind. It may have been a break-through in bad judgment, but had nothing of scientific distinction about it.

For the moment, let us leave aside the problems of the forty-year-old in my clinic and consider the treatment of very much older women. The truth is that with the use of donor eggs, taken from the ovaries of younger women, it is perfectly possible to get any human female pregnant, be she seventy years old or merely seven. If the woman in question is menopausal, then she will no longer have eggs in her ovaries. Also, she will no longer be producing much of the female hormone, oestrogen. Oestrogen is the hormone, also produced from the ovaries, which gives the characteristic shape to the female body and which initiates and maintains breast development. It also ensures that the uterus grows to its full size and is capable of carrying a baby. Oestrogen produces the growth of the uterine lining, the endometrium, giving rise to regular periods when it is shed each month. Girls before puberty and women after the menopause do not have periods because they lack this hormone. No matter what age, any female when given oestrogen artificially by mouth or by injection can be brought to a state of potential child-bearing. With the simple transfer of a donor egg, fertilised outside the body by IVF, to the primed uterus, pregnancy can ensue. Once the pregnancy is established, it will produce enough hormone itself from its placenta for the safe maintenance of the pregnancy.

This then is the much vaunted 'breakthrough', widely heralding Dr Antinori and similar colleagues in the less discerning press. Admittedly, not even Dr Antinori has recommended this treatment for schoolchildren who want a baby. The question really is whether or not such treatments are justified in women who are well past their natural menopause.

The reason why I am so critical of these treatments is partly because I think we may run the risk of blurring the medical arguments against them, because of sympathy towards older 'desperate' women, or possibly because of baser, commercial motives. It seems to me that there are very good reasons why treating women in their late fifties or early sixties is undesirable, and potentially very harmful.

First is concern for the woman herself. Pregnancy and childbirth, not to say early child nurture, are demanding for all parents, but obviously more burdensome for the woman. Statistics show that maternal deaths are much more likely in pregnant women in later childbearing years. A forty-plus-year-old has a tenfold increased risk of death in pregnancy compared with a woman in her twenties. This is not such a great risk, admittedly, because death associated with pregnancy is nowadays a very rare event. Nevertheless, this risk will be higher still in a woman of fifty or sixty. More to the point, the risk is not only that of death, but a more general and important one of serious ill-health.

The risk of high blood pressure and hence toxaemia of pregnancy are much more likely in women bearing children in their later years. Diabetes, too, is much more likely because of the strain that pregnancy puts on the metabolic system in the body. These diseases of pregnancy are not only dangerous for the mother – frequently necessitating prolonged hospital care – and possibly irreversibly damaging health, they also affect the developing infant. All older pregnant mothers are prone to give birth to small, growth-retarded babies; this risk will be greater should a serious disease of pregnancy occur. Consequently, there will be a greater risk of loss of the baby after delivery. Incidentally, it is now quite well known that all IVF babies are at slightly greater risk of mishap during pregnancy and delivery – death rates are higher after IVF – and this risk to the infant will be accentuated in older mothers.

Other physical risks to the older mother include heart disease, particularly heart attacks. This is because, after the menopause, a woman's arteries start to harden and she develops the same risk of coronary thrombosis as a man. Treatment with oestrogens on a short-term basis – for example, to get a woman pregnant – will not reverse this process, and the immense increase in the blood volume and extra work the heart has to do during pregnancy make a risk of heart attack very real. Another potential killer is venous thrombosis. Older women are much more prone to develop blood clots in the veins. Occasionally, these blood clots can become dislodged by mere movement of the body and block off the blood supply to a lung; this can cause sudden death by pulmonary embolus. A blood clot can also enter the circulation of the brain and cause a stroke. Both these risks are more likely in any woman who has had an operative delivery such as a Caesarean section; it is relevant here to observe that older pregnant patients are three times more likely to need a Caesarean section.

In order to get the older patient pregnant 'at all costs', many units outside Britain transfer many embryos to the uterus. This practice is banned by the HFEA and in the UK the maximum permitted number of embryos is three, irrespective of the mother's age. Regrettably this has not prevented at least one British doctor opening a satellite clinic overseas, in a country where regulation on such matters is absent, and richer patients over the age of forty may travel there. The risk is, of course, of multiple pregnancy. A pregnancy with a single baby is complicated enough for an older woman, but twins make the risks of serious complications of pregnancy much more likely. It would be unusual for an older woman with a twin pregnancy not to require prolonged time in hospital, and premature birth, miscarriage, or babies which do not survive will be a common event. Unfortunately, with more than two embryos there is an undoubted risk of triplets or of a higher order multiple pregnancy. The risks then become very serious. Hospital care from about six months of pregnancy (if the pregnancy survives that long) is highly probable. Premature delivery, usually by complicated Caesarean section, is certain. Severely growth-retarded babies, if they live at all, will usually be delivered, and of course such babies may suffer permanent effects throughout their life.

In order to get around these serious obstetric problems, some clinics, particularly in the USA, suggest multiple embryo transfer to these older women, followed by the offer of selective fetal reduction. Selective reduction is the destruction of 'surplus' fetuses, usually by passing a needle into the heart or the sac of fluid around the fetus and injecting some embryo-toxic material. Generally speaking such manoeuvres have to be delayed until after the eighth week of pregnancy, which in itself is highly emotionally charged for the patient. Leaving aside the issue of whether it is morally right to wantonly induce life and then destroy it in this way, and leaving aside any judgment regarding abortion, this is a reprehensible and pernicious practice. Selective termination risks loss of the whole pregnancy if things go wrong. The idea that doctors could risk the emotional state of their patients in this way seems to me to be frightening. A desperate woman finds herself pregnant only to find that, once the pregnancy is established, it is lost. Moreover, it has been lost with her consent and connivance, no matter how reluctant. Even if the pregnancy is not lost and a single baby or twins survive, most women will experience a grief reaction of varying severity over the loss of the other babies. Moreover, it would not be unusual for any guilt feeling about the reduction to manifest itself, after birth, in rejection of the child that arbitrarily was chosen for survival. Doctors tamper with these powerful emotions at the peril of others.

Even so, these various arguments and the physical risks of pregnancy to a much older woman seem to me to be relatively less important. After all, if a woman has first been fully informed about them, acknowledges their existence and gives consent for treatment to get pregnant, surely the doctor is simply respecting his patient's autonomy by helping her? As it happens, there is, I believe, a different kind of medical risk. In many of these cases there is a much more serious risk of psychological or emotional damage. In order to understand this, we need to consider why women in

IVF in Older Women

their late fifties or early sixties might feel such desperation for a child, at almost any cost. There is considerable evidence that many such women are actually going through a protracted bereavement process, mourning not only their lack of a child but also the aging process which brings with it inability to procreate. Such a pronounced grief reaction can result in a huge emotional backlash if things go wrong. When such a woman finally, possibly after much persuasion, manages to find a doctor who is prepared to treat her, she is buoyed up with even more fraught emotions. She enters the hurdle race of IVF, with the probable outcome of failure. Any underlying state of depression or grief surfaces once again, but in a much more intense form. Worse still, a grieving woman in this situation becomes pregnant, but miscarries – an outcome which, in any case, is more likely in older women. The shock of such an event in a woman who is already disturbed or depressed can be catastrophic. I have seen this reaction twice in women in their forties, and it was a horrendous experience not only for them, but also for their close family and for us doctors who had reluctantly gone along with treatment feeling vaguely that psychological problems could occur. One of these women committed suicide by swallowing weed-killer – which led to a short, severe, fulminating illness before her death from kidney and liver failure. Another woman attempted suicide twice, but her attempts at self-destruction were intercepted by her distraught husband. She then had an acute psychotic illness akin to schizophrenia, hearing voices and repeatedly having visions of herself as the Virgin Mary. She was committed to a mental hospital and was released after eighteen weeks but never recovered her previous vivacious and attractive personality. Although the risk of such severe derangement or self-inflicted damage is unlikely after IVF treatment, it is clear that this is not a risk for which a patient can legitimately give 'informed' consent beforehand.

Many people have argued also that the treatment of older mothers is not in the interest of the child. An older woman, it is stated, will have much less energy to devote both to pregnancy and subsequently to caring for the baby. The chore of getting up for night feeds, of being on call throughout the day, and the constant attention that a growing toddler needs as he or she explores their surroundings, place considerable demands on parents. A woman giving birth at sixty will be seventy years old before the child is even a teenager, by which time the child is not unlikely to be an orphan. The embarrassment of children of much younger elderly parents at being taken to school by their 'grandmother' is well documented. Such a child, not likely to be an only child in view of parental infertility, will be denied much of the usual physical stimulus that is the prerogative of normal childhood. Parents in their seventies are unlikely to be adequate goalkeepers in the back garden.

One frequently heard argument in favour of treating older women is that not to do so is in some way sexist. Men are fertile well into their seventies; Picasso was a father when over eighty. There is surely, though, a difference between male and female parenting. This is not a sexist attitude, but in most societies, certainly in our so-called advanced Western society, the female partner generally plays a much more crucial role in rearing children.

One of the serious arguments against treating post-menopausal women in this way that is seldom heard concerns the views of the donor. As we have seen, a woman who is post-menopausal can only conceive if she receives an egg from another woman. Compared to post-menopausal recipients, donors are much younger women. In England, by regulation they have to be under 35 years old, mostly to reduce any risk of a genetic defect such as Down's syndrome in any resulting child. Donors go through considerable inconvenience and some risk to donate their eggs, which are, of course, their own unique genetic material. What rights should they have in deciding who gets this precious gift? Currently it seems that they have none. This is a problem because the recruitment of egg donors is, as discussed earlier, very difficult. Their motivation has to be very strong to go through the arduous process that egg donation involves. They need to feel that they are helping a desperate, infertile woman, with whose feelings they can strongly relate. They are mostly women who have been very committed to, and very rewarded by, motherhood themselves. Not surprisingly, in view of the background to their altruism, they usually express a strong desire that any child that is born (who after all is genetically theirs) is brought up in a stable and good relationship. Their act of donation is, psychologically at least, not without strings.

My contact with prospective donors has made it clear to me that they generally expect no control over any child that may be produced, and seldom show any wish for contact. However, they usually do evince interest in whether their actions have resulted in success – a pregnancy. They are also frequently concerned that their child is in 'a good home' and will be happy. Whenever we at Hammersmith have asked potential donors whether they might have any objections to their eggs going to a woman in her later fifties, they have usually shown fairly extreme concern. In this country, it certainly seems that altruistic donors see their eggs going to women with whom they can identify closely, and to potential families similar to their own ideals.

Whether or not donors have some rights with regard to the way in which their eggs are 'distributed', it is clear that altruistic women will be much less likely to go through the complexities of the donation procedure if they are unhappy about the recipients of their generosity. Pure pragmatism argues that doctors should be cautious about who receives donated eggs, otherwise supplies may dry up. There is evidence for this from what is already happening in the USA. Considerable press publicity was given to an IVF clinic in New York City, and another clinic in Los Angeles. Both clinics had made a considerable 'reputation' treating postmenopausal women using donated eggs. Neither clinic was reticent about its treatment and featured prominently on television and in the newspapers. In the commercial atmosphere that surrounds certain aspects of American medical care, it is not necessarily to the financial disadvantage of a private clinic (and in the US, even the university clinics are run on a private basis) to be prominent in the media. Great publicity was given to the policy of treating older women, but the supply of altruistic donors from the general public dried up almost totally. Any eggs now used in most donor programmes in the US are so-called 'spare' eggs from other IVF patients' treatment cycles.

All this raises the reason for what I feel is my most powerful objection to treating women who are well over the age of fifty. Most members of the public think it a misuse of technology, or even find it distasteful or possibly abhorrent. Whether or not they are right to feel as they do is, in a sense, irrelevant. When at the cutting edge of any new technology, its protagonists must take public opinion into account when considering what is ethical and therefore acceptable. IVF is a privileged and precious technology, poorly funded and, at the moment, largely the province of people who are somewhat financially better off than average. It is also a powerful technology, at the very cutting edge of what is possible in medicine. It has a great potential for human good, particularly as we unravel some of the mysteries of human genetics. To bring it into public disrepute would be to jeopardise that powerful but delicate technology. What limited funding is available may dry up, and important research on the very beginnings of human life might be curtailed. That would be too high a price to pay for the right to treat a few older women whose right to this risky therapy is arguable at best.

There is also an interesting medical principle here. It is the issue of when a treatment ceases to be for medical reasons, and is being used for social ones. Most people would have little concern over treating young women with a premature menopause which has been brought on by cancer treatment (as in the case of Rebecca). The use of donor eggs in these cases, as it is in young women whose ovaries just stop functioning in their twenties or thirties, seems quite justified. When we treat such women, we are treating them for what is clearly defined as a pathological and therefore 'unnatural' condition. It seems to me that women in their fifties or sixties, though, are not having treatment for a diseased state, but rather for social reasons. Indeed, there almost seems a consumerist attitude about some of these requests. It is as if the baby is some kind of commodity that is being procured like any other 'article' which is wanted. It is not irrelevant that, almost exclusively, the women being treated in very much later life are those who are prepared to pay quite large sums of money to have their dreams fulfilled. It is perhaps interesting to speculate whether the fulfilment of those dreams is actually bringing happiness to those aging women and their children. Here is an area absolutely rich for sociologists to research.

However, in spite of all the publicity which leads people to believe perhaps that there is a glut of elderly ladies seeking pregnancy, very few women well past the normal menopause actually appear to seek this treatment. At Hammersmith, in the last five years we cannot find one application for a woman over the age of fifty-one seeking fertility treatment. The oldest we have actually treated was forty-nine, and then only with her own eggs. Information from the two largest clinics in this country known to have a permissive attitude to egg donation for much older women, leads me to believe that there are probably fewer than twenty requests annually in the UK. Almost certainly, some of these women would have contacted all the major units in hope of treatment, so the figure of twenty is likely to be an overestimate. The big problem really exists for those women approaching their menopause, the women in the age range thirty-eight to forty-eight years old, for whom fertility is declining naturally at a rapid pace. They are not seeking egg donation because they are still producing their own eggs, although possibly not very efficiently.

The main problem is that these older women find it difficult to get treatment at all. We saw in Chapter 1 how a woman from Sheffield was refused IVF treatment because she was thirty-seven years old. The implication was that it was not worth offering her treatment because she was now too old. Treatment would be less likely to work and therefore the NHS funding health authority would not be getting good value for its money. This seems a very hard argument. There will be many infertile women at thirty-seven who will be extremely likely to get pregnant with IVF. Indeed, there are many women in their early forties (with for example blocked tubes) who will be more fertile with IVF than a woman with a similar condition in her twenties. The chance of pregnancy will depend on how responsive the ovaries are and how good are the eggs which are produced with stimulation. The increasing subfertility with age only reflects what happens on average, and individual women may well do better than the average. Not all of us are 5 feet 10 inches (1.75 metres) in height.

It certainly seems ironic that the patient in her late thirties or early forties should be discriminated against by the NHS in this way. She has delayed childbearing until she has developed a skill, and possibly a career. She is likely to be more mature, possibly even a better parent. By being in employment she has contributed to the economy and now that she wants to start her family, she is told that the economic climate within the health service is such that her treatment is not affordable.

What is clear is that wanting to get pregnant and being in late reproductive years is a desperate situation for many infertile women. I am often in the position of conducting a clinic in which nearly all the patients are over forty. They exhibit all the sadness of infertility and all its problems, but often in the most extreme form. They are often going through quite severe grief, and feel angry and guilty. Many of these couples, particularly the women, who perceive themselves as getting older, are very prepared to gamble almost anything on getting pregnant. They are extraordinarily vulnerable because they are prepared to try almost anything. I think this is why I get so angry with doctors such as Dr Antinori in Italy, who are prepared to try to 'help' these sad women with sometimes preposterous efforts to get them a pregnancy. They are ripe for exploitation, and we professionals have to show extreme care and sensitivity about how we handle their problem. To 'give hope' may sound a wonderful approach but it is fraught with danger, particularly when hope is dashed afterwards. Infertility treatment is always worth considering, but it is not worth doing at all costs.

Chapter Seven

Developing the Future

In the previous chapter, I described how by removing a cell from the embryo and analysing the DNA or the chromosomes, we could get some idea of its health. The problem with that test is that it requires an operation to remove a cell. It is what is referred to medically as an invasive test. Clearly, if non-invasive testing were available, it would be better to use it. Any investigation which is invasive does carry more significant implications. The embryo may not be sacrosanct, but it should surely be regarded as worthy of all reasonable protection possible. For this reason, the idea of non-invasive testing was extremely attractive to our team and we have spent many years developing some techniques to try this.

There are excellent reasons for wanting to assess the general viability of an embryo before it is placed in the uterus. As we have seen, only 20% of human embryos are capable of becoming a baby. More than one embryo is transferred to the uterus to improve the chance of IVF working; this of course also increases the chance of multiple birth. Some years ago, Henry Leese from York University, devised a method for potentially assessing the viability of mouse embryos, and he helped us to develop the test which we use in human embryos. Hours after fertilisation, the embryo is placed in a tiny droplet of fluid so small it can only just be seen with the naked eye. The droplet together with the embryo in it are placed under a special silicone oil which isolates it from the atmosphere. The dish is then returned to an incubator at body temperature. The fluid contains a known concentration of sugar, either a sugar called pyruvate or glucose, both of which are consumed by embryos. After a measured interval of time, say up to twenty-four hours,

Developing the Future

the embryo is removed from its droplet, and placed in another droplet and the process can be repeated. The little droplets of fluid in which the embryos have grown are not thrown away. On the contrary, they are really precious. Using a special machine, the droplets can be quickly analysed to see how much of the original sugar is missing – this is the amount used by the embryo. The amount of sugar used gives the amount of energy that it has used. Embryos which use more energy are more metabolically active and, in theory, are more likely to be viable.

This test was extensively researched in our lab by Kate Hardy and a PhD student, Joe Conaghan. Kate is one of the most organised scientists I know. She, more than anyone else, has been responsible for the degree of meticulous administration in our lab. She is quite giggly, blonde and beautiful and has an excellent mind, which she tries to hide. Kate cannot bear chaos and is always busy, gently organising people, whether it is for trips punting in Cambridge, her old university, or making sure they wash up their laboratory apparatus – she is really like A.A. Milne's Rabbit. I have only seen her totally fazed once, when I told her that I was bored seeing patients all the time and was intending to come into the lab to do my own experiments. The tan from her recent skiing trip faded: 'Oh Robert, we'll never find anything again'.

The metabolic test on embryos works but, as yet, is not sufficiently discriminatory to be really useful and to pick consistently the viable embryos for IVF treatments. Amongst other projects, Kate is now working on improvements of this test. In particular, she is looking to see how embryos take up amino acids. These are the substances which go to make proteins, and we feel that if we can work out how rapidly the embryo is using protein, we shall have a better assessment of its viability. Another important reason for continuing with these non-invasive tests is that by looking, for example, at how embryos grow in different concentrations of sugars, we can work out the best composition for the culture medium we use. There is no doubt that Kate's experiments have added to our knowledge of how to improve the environment of embryos. With the knowledge we have gained from our sugar droplets, we have adjusted both the sugar concentration and the amount of certain amino acids in our culture fluids. The result has been a definite improvement in embryo growth.

Clearly under law there is no problem about the ethicality of doing the kind of work with which Kate is involved. It is helping to improve infertility treatment, allowable by the 1990 Act of Parliament. However, things are not always that clear cut. When embryo research was originally considered by Parliament, it was decided that research would be allowable to:

a promote advances in the treatment of infertility;
b increase knowledge about the causes of congenital disease;
c increase knowledge about the causes of miscarriage;
d develop more effective techniques of contraception;
e develop methods for detecting the presence of gene or chromosome abnormalities in embryos before implantation, *'or more generally for the purpose of increasing knowledge about the creation and development of embryos and enabling such knowledge to be applied'*. This last part of the sentence implies some commitment to basic research, but literally only where it has the goal of being applied for some good purpose. What about research for which there is no clear evidence that it has applicable value?

For some time now we have been interested in one of the most basic of mechanisms. All the genes are present from the time of fertilisation, but they do not necessarily function immediately. The volumes of the book of life are printed in the DNA, but the DNA is not read or 'transcribed'. Transcription occurs at a later stage when the DNA forms the template for the messenger RNA, which leaves the nucleus – the bookcase – to enter the cytoplasm of the cell. There it gives the instructions to make the specific protein which produces a particular characteristic. In the previous chapter, I compared the genes to entries in an encyclopaedia. Some of these entries, this information, will be used every day of life, other entries may only be read occasionally or even just once. Immediately after fertilisation, most of the genetic activity does not come from the embryo at all, but from the egg. The maternal messenger RNA is still present from the cytoplasm of the egg. This regulates most of the basic functions of the first few cells in the embryo until the embryonic genes are switched on. At first, only basic housekeeping genes, entries which are read every day, are switched on. These are the genes which, for example, regulate cell division and the basic use of nutrients (like Kate's sugars) in the cell. It is only later that specific genes which have a less general function will start to express. For example, dystrophin is a normal protein important for muscle function. Without it the muscle does not contract properly. When the gene that codes for dystrophin is abnormal (there is a misprint in the encyclopaedia entry) the normal dystrophin protein is not made and the person suffers from muscular dystrophy. The embryo carries the abnormal dystrophin gene from the moment of fertilisation but it does not yet suffer from muscular dystrophy because the gene product, the dystrophin, is not made until the muscle tissues are being formed.

In the past it has generally been assumed that genes do not switch on until there is a specific need for their product. We have looked at one set of genes, the genes which determine sex. Dr Asangla Ao, one of the scientists on the team, and Pierre Ray, another postgraduate scientist studying for his PhD, developed methods for detecting the messenger RNA produced by the sex-determining genes. These genes, which are on the Y chromosome, are the genes which produce male characteristics. The sex-determining genes can be identified using PCR which, as I have already described, is an exquisitely sensitive process, very subject to contamination. Identification of the transcript, the messenger RNA, is very much harder. The RNA has essentially a similar structure to the DNA, so a modification of the PCR technique can be used, but it requires the most meticulous approach. Until very recently, it was quite impossible to detect the RNA in just a single cell. This meant that, in order to get enough RNA to measure, Asangla and Pierre had to take several embryo cells for the test to work. As there are only one or two cells soon after fertilisation in each embryo, they had to pool several embryos to get a result. To our real surprise, sex-determining genes produce their RNA within a few hours of fertilisation. There seems no reason for this because obviously at this stage and for some days to come the embryo is just a clump of totally undifferentiated cells. The fact that the genes are starting to produce their message this early is very interesting, but completely useless, information.

About the time we were doing the gene expression experiments there was some news from the USA which suggested that in cattle, the male embryos were slightly bigger than females at a similar time after fertilisation. This did not make any sense to us and we rather ignored this information. However, a friend of ours, Dr Gene Pergament from Chicago, published his findings following a trawl through the results of his local IVF unit. From the IVF clinic records, he checked the number of cells in each human embryo on the day of transfer, which in this clinic was always on the second day after fertilisation. Then he correlated these findings with the sex of any baby born. What he found made him very excited, namely that embryos which had more cells and were further advanced in development at the time of transfer tended to be boys.

We found Gene Pergament's news very difficult to believe. The idea that boy embryos might be bigger than girl embryos so soon after fertilisation seemed extraordinarily unlikely. With considerable scepticism we looked at the embryo data from the Hammersmith programme to try to disprove the message we were getting from Gene. Amazingly, our data tended to fall in line with his findings; the male embryos were indeed slightly more advanced in development.

So if males were slightly more advanced in development, it could follow they were more active metabolically – using more energy. With this idea, our team decided to use the non-invasive sugar test. A series of embryos was placed in the tiny sugar droplets. At day 1, day 2 and day 3 after fertilisation, the droplets were tested to see how much sugar had been consumed. Then another member of the team, who did not know the results of the work and therefore could not influence the findings, used our method of DNA analysis to identify the sex of each of the embryos. The results clearly showed that males consume 20% more sugar than females. It appears that we men are more aggressive from the moment of fertilisation.

This may seem like useless information. Indeed, had we only been doing goal-orientated research we would not have gone down this route at all. But a very interesting thought now struck us. Figures from around the world show that, after natural conception, more boys are born than girls. The ratio is roughly 51:49. This is such a consistent finding that it cannot be due to chance. If the sex of human babies was completely a matter of random chance, with the 100 million births each year in the world, the figures would balance out and should be virtually precisely 50:50. But the proportion of males is always slightly greater.

With this knowledge we have started to analyse the ratio of male to female embryos after fertilisation in the IVF programme. Obviously we cannot sex most of the embryos and the data are nowhere near complete, but preliminary findings suggest that quite a few more female embryos may be formed initially, even though the birth ratio is roughly even. What we may possibly be seeing with the increased metabolism is a genetic adjustment. Perhaps the male embryos may have to be more active to be more viable; this increases their chance of implantation and hence roughly maintains the correct ratio between the sexes. I find this information interesting because it has been known for some years that outside influences in some other species may alter the ratio between males and females. Turtles and tortoises can change the sex of their offspring by altering the temperature at which their eggs are incubated. With eggs kept up to 28°C, all the babies are males; above 32°C and all are females.

What is particularly fascinating is that there are times when the ratio between the births of males to females changes in the human population. There is some evidence that after some major disasters, for example, an increased number of males are born. This phenomenon has been documented for over 100 years, since Dr Ploss in Austria showed in 1882 that more male babies were born when there had been a recent war or some natural calamity. There is evidence also that for a time after the First World War when so many young men were killed, there was an excess number of male births in Europe. It is interesting to speculate that this is an example of where human genes may be influenced by environmental conditions. Perhaps our studies on the stage of growth when human sex-determining genes are switched on is not so pointless after all. If for some reason, perhaps an environmental one, they are switched on a little later, a different proportion of male

Developing the Future

to female embryos may implant. This would be one of a number of ways with which humans could unwittingly control the sex of their babies.

Asangla Ao is a very laid-back individual and we really only got to discuss all these results at a team ski-trip. As I mentioned before, for some time now it has been my pleasure to go skiing with about a dozen members of the team. I learn most of my science then. The first time Asangla joined the team ski-trip she was given her air-ticket, but did not appear at Heathrow Airport at 7.30 in the morning. Frantic calls were made but we could not locate her. Finally, in great disappointment the rest of us got onto the plane. After we arrived in Switzerland, it transpired that on the way to the airport, Asangla (who has an Indian passport and had never previously gone skiing) found that she had got the wrong visa after queuing the day before at the *Swedish* embassy. She arrived at the chalet at about 1 o'clock the following morning and seemed totally unperturbed. She was, however, rather more excited about the gene expression work.

One of the implications of our work on detecting the sex of an embryo is that it could be used for a very accurate method of sex selection. We have already used it for that purpose, of course, in the case of sex-linked genetic disorders, transferring only those embryos identified as female in families at risk of having children with haemophilia or muscular dystrophy. Humans have chased the possibility of choosing the sex of their child since earliest recorded history. In general, there has always been a preference for male children. Ancient Greece may have been the cradle of modern democracy but even there, in that apparently enlightened civilisation, women had no more than the status of slaves. Greek philosophers such as Empedocles and Aristotle showed unusual interest in ways of manipulating the sex of a baby, and Hippocrates, the father of medicine, thought that intercourse lying on one's right side would produce boys. Female infanticide was certainly practised in ancient Sparta and, remarkably, even to this day the sacrifice of female infants is not unknown. In a speech to the United Nations Conference on Women in 1995, Prime Minister Benazir Bhutto of Pakistan said 'Girl children are often abandoned or aborted...boys are wanted because their worth is considered more than that of a girl.' This speech was given in Peking; although the sex ratio is naturally around 106:100 in most parts of the world, in China it is 114:100. Here, as in parts of India and elsewhere in Asia, ultrasound is used to detect the sex of a baby during pregnancy, and late termination is considered if the male genitalia cannot be visualised on the ultrasound screen. This shocking practice makes it clear that any method of selecting male children might be exploited in some societies.

It has been widely suggested that there would be little harm done if our method of sex selection was used for those families who want a balance in the sex ratio in their own offspring. At first glance, it seems perfectly reasonable to agree to offer a male embryo transfer to a family already 'afflicted' with three daughters. Indeed, it has been said that such a child, born after sex selection might feel especially wanted. What little harm in that? There is, in my view, more potential harm than might be first thought. In treating a child as a commodity in this way, other siblings may be devalued. Alternatively, the selected child may not reach parental expectations in other ways. On the whole, it seems to me to be probably the wrong reason to have a child.

At Hammersmith, we have never considered undertaking sex selection for social reasons, and have used our technique strictly to combat severe inherited diseases. There have, however, been one or two extraordinary and superficially tempting opportunities. Once, I received a phone call one afternoon asking me to stand by later that week for a telephone conversation with the agent of an 'important person' in a large country in the Middle East. Two days later the call came and I was asked whether I would be prepared to undertake male sex selection for the employer of this 'important person'. I said firmly that I would not countenance this. I was then told that the Ruler of this country would esteem it an especial favour and that I could expect a reward. I said that it would not be legal to do this because British regulations were opposed to sex selection. The agent said that it would be simple to do it in his country where there were no legal problems. I pointed out that I would have to fly my team of eight people to his country to do this. I was immediately told that there would be no problem about this and I was offered a personal fee of £20,000. I replied that the Ruler should be told that he might get rather poor medicine if the doctors he was employing were prepared to bend their principles for money. My torturer rang off, and I considered this the end of the matter. Two days later my phone went again. The persistent agent told me that he was now empowered to offer me a personal fee of £50,000. I asked if he thought this improved fee would improve the quality of the medicine, and politely told him that we were not prepared to jeopardise the reputation of a vulnerable branch of medicine and that I hoped this would be the end of the matter. Two days later he rang me to ask if I would recommend another doctor who would be prepared to carry out the treatment!

In Chapter Four, Embryo Research, I examined how research on the human embryo had been developed to start to improve our ability to prevent genetic diseases, and some of the ethical issues involved in this work. There have now been preliminary attempts to prevent serious gene defects like cystic fibrosis, and some of the sex-linked disorders. Work to prevent chromosomal problems such as Down's syndrome and some of the disorders connected with repeated miscarriage has also started to produce tentative results. Around the world a number of diseases have now been screened for in embryos and, apart from those already discussed, they include some of the blood disorders which cause a massive number of deaths annually. Moreover, such diseases have major economic implications for the countries where they are prevalent. For example, in Thailand well over 100,000 babies die each year from thalassaemia. It is not just the death rate, but the fact that surviving children need blood transfusions every three or four weeks if they are to have any chance of reasonable health, and the financial pressures on those families carrying these gene defects and on the State, which provides some care, are huge.

But one of the unresolved questions is where do we draw a line? Which diseases constitute such a threat to a person, that it is justified to use these complex and currently expensive technologies? We have already started to scratch the surface of this hugely difficult ethical problem with our attempts at screening embryos for Down's syndrome. As it happens, generally there has not been much criticism of this work because termination of pregnancy is already widely undertaken for pregnancies with Down's syndrome. Abortion for this condition is broadly accepted in most European countries, and is legal under the 1967 Act of Parliament.

Down's syndrome is caused by three copies of chromosome 21 in each cell nucleus. It was first recognised as a clinical disease as long ago as 1846, when it was seen as being associated with what was then called 'idiocy'. In 1866, Dr Langdon Down (hence the name of the disease) described its characteristics fairly comprehensively and called it 'Mongolian idiocy' because of the curious facial appearance of babies with it. Their face is round and flat, and the eyes appear slightly slit-like. The nose is short and upturned, and the tongue frequently protrudes. Nowadays, the term 'Mongolism' is properly criticised because of its racial

Developing the Future

overtones. Ironically, the cause of Down's syndrome was first discovered by Dr Lejeune in 1959. Professor Lejeune has a distinguished reputation as a geneticist. He described the three copies of chromosome 21 which give rise to the disease. I say ironically because his description led to the method of antenatal diagnosis of the disease and hence to doctors' ability to offer abortion to women who carry an affected baby. It so happens that Professor Lejeune is an orthodox Roman Catholic, and I understand that his discovery and the uses to which it has been put have caused him great pain. Certainly, when there were attempts to ban embryo research in this country, Professor Lejeune repeatedly flew over from Paris in an effort to support proposals by 'Right to Life' groups to halt our work.

Down's syndrome occurs about 1 in every 700 births. Being a relatively 'minor' chromosomal defect, it is compatible with life, though many fetuses with it undoubtedly abort spontaneously. It affects male babies slightly more frequently than females, and is commoner in the pregnancies of older women (Chapter Six, IVF in Older Women). The chances of it occurring may also be slightly influenced by the age of the father, though this is still controversial scientifically.

Down's syndrome babies tend to be smaller than average, and are often born prematurely. They tend to be 'floppy' at birth, feed poorly, are very sleepy and unresponsive to stimuli. As they grow, their faces show signs of premature aging, yet their physical development is retarded. Generally they do not sit up until a year old and cannot walk until two years. The major feature of their condition is the mental retardation which is variable but can frequently be severe. A typical IQ may be 40, but in some children it is as high as 70. A normal kindergarten environment is extremely important if they are to be stimulated intellectually at all. Early institutionalisation is undoubtedly the worst thing for these children. However, by the age of seven, it becomes impossible to maintain these children in normal schools, because they tire quickly and are unstable. They also become aware of their own mental handicap. Probably by then they should attend special day schools, but after adolescence their care presents a real problem. Obviously care may be much easier in a person with an IQ of 70 than 30, but one of the problems is that the degree of mental retardation is unpredictable. In addition to the retardation, about half of Down's sufferers have a serious heart defect and death frequently occurs when surgical attempts are made at correction. They frequently have serious, even fatal, malformations of the bowel, problems with their teeth, damage and deformity of the spine and joints, and damaged eye sight which is of course difficult to correct with glasses in someone who is severely mentally retarded. Sometimes blindness occurs. Down's syndrome children have a high likelihood of serious chest infections which often cause death, and their immunity is less adequate than in normal people. They frequently suffer from unpleasant itchy and unsightly skin diseases. They also have a very much increased risk (about twenty-fold) of developing leukaemia, compared with normal children. About one-fifth of these children die by about the age of five from a variety of causes, and about one-quarter to one-third by twenty-five.

I have described Down's syndrome to a fairly full degree quite deliberately. Clearly it is fully compatible with life in some cases, and many parents report how happy their Down's syndrome children are. It is definitely not invariably fatal, but the quality of life is undoubtedly impaired severely and in most cases very severely. It is sometimes argued that doctors want to persuade mothers with abnormal pregnancies like this of the virtues of termination of pregnancy. But this is not a fair assessment. Most of the pressure undoubtedly comes from prospective parents, not from society, nor medical and nursing advisers. If antenatal screening is to be used at all, patients must be protected to ensure their freedom to use these screening techniques. Consequently they should not be routine, and certainly not without informed consent.

Some patients who have one Down's baby decide against termination. Because there is a slight risk of the condition repeating itself in a subsequent pregnancy, they then conceive a second affected pregnancy. Nearly all the mothers that I have come across then decide that they will have an abortion. I make no judgment about this but it seems to me that, from an absolutist point of view, there is no moral difference between the decision in terminating the first and terminating the second pregnancy. Here it seems to me is a situation where the autonomy of the parents has ultimately to be respected, and finally it is their choice which decides the issue.

As preimplantation genetic diagnosis gains in impetus, it is argued that governments might decide to put pressure on women known to carry these genetic defects to have this kind of reproductive screening. The suggestion has been that people refusing screening might face financial penalties, for example. This seems rather unlikely. If governments were so heavy-handed, it is far more likely that there would be pressure to have antenatal diagnosis and termination of pregnancy. This would certainly be cheaper, though of course research into IVF may reduce the cost of embryo screening. Potential political inter-ference with human reproduction would be an extremely deficient reason to halt the work we are doing. Rather we should ensure that society accepts that the right of individuals to use or not to use prenatal and preimplant-ation diagnosis should be protected.

John Robertson, the American lawyer, has written that 'although abortion may be a symbolic devaluation of human life, these symbolic losses can be justified by the burdens on the woman who chooses to abort. Faced with an unwanted pregnancy, abortion offers her relief from the burdens of unwanted gestation and child rearing. On this argument, her freedom from those burdens trumps the symbolic cost of ending a fetus's life.' Certainly, if we believe that the fetus is more valuable and deserving of protection than the early preimplantation embryo, then what Robertson says about abortion certainly would apply to our use of IVF technology. However, there is still a major dilemma here when we consider the possibility of less life-threatening conditions rather than fatal diseases or conditions such as Down's syndrome, whose impact can place a huge burden on parents.

Our work in embryonic genetic diagnosis is about to explore more controversial areas. There are a number of single-gene defects which cause cancer; if one of these genes is carried, there is the strong likelihood that the carrier may develop cancer. This probability may be as high as 90% and, moreover, the cancer usually occurs at a fairly early age, mostly in young adulthood. It is also relevant that many of these inherited cancers tend to cause tumours which are not infrequently difficult to treat. An inherited cancer is likely to cause death in most cases in spite of sometimes prolonged treatment and considerable suffering. One such typical cancer is caused by the BRCA1 gene. Women with this gene carry a 90% probability of developing breast cancer, mostly before the age of thirty-five. Males with this gene appear not to be at risk.

I have one patient, a carrier of this gene, who had both breasts removed at the age of thirty, as a prophylactic measure in case the disease might develop in future. She has had six members of her immediate family develop the disease, five of whom died by the age of forty – two under thirty years old. She has used contraception since marriage and came requesting selection of a male embryo after IVF, on the grounds that a boy could not develop the disease. If when her son grew up he passed this gene on to one of his children (it is carried on chromosome 17 so there is a 50:50 chance of this), by that time, she reckoned, there would be better treatment or a cure. As it happens, her specific gene has now been sequenced, so I suggested to her that we try to identify the actual gene in her embryo using PCR rather than just use sexing. This would of course eliminate that gene from future generations. We do not have ethical approval for this as yet, so I have made a written application to our hospital's ethics committee and should hear soon whether this will be sanctioned. Once I have the permission from them, I still need to apply to the regulatory HFEA before I do the treatment. There are a number of similar 'cancer' genes. One causes familial polyposis and, in a family at risk, will affect 50% of its members. Death from colon cancer is likely; one patient we have seen from Newcastle has had seven of her family affected. Other cancers which are genetically determined in this way include retinoblastoma, which affects the brain of young children, endocrine neoplasia, which causes generally widespread cancer for which a cure is very unlikely because of rapid spread of the disease, and some forms of usually fatal kidney cancer.

The treatment of these diseases by embryo selection certainly goes beyond Robertson's criteria of 'a burden on the pregnant or child-rearing woman'. These diseases are manifest a long time after normal maternal responsibility. They affect young adults who, before they die, may contribute to society in a most important way. Wolfgang Amadeus Mozart was thirty-five when he died in 1791; Franz Schubert thirty-one when he died in 1828. Had their embryos been discarded for some reason, their lives and creativity would have been lost to the world.

Nor could one say that embryos carrying these genes have been harmed by being born. They have no way of being born free of their gene defect at present, unless of course we could do gene therapy in the embryo – not a possible medical option at the moment. Conditions such as adult cancers, no matter how horrible or unsuccessful the treatment, do not make a child's life so appalling or anxious that its interests are best served by not being born. This is the very argument used in reverse to demonstrate why society cannot justify a coercive policy towards sterilisation or contraception for the parents of such children.

All this is clearly why doctors like myself must apply for ethical approval for complex issues of this kind. The constitution of ethics committees with the heavy involvement of lay individuals probably does remain the best protection that society has against wrong decisions by individual scientists and doctors. As we have seen, their decisions are by no means infallible, but they provide an important interface with society. As it happens, I strongly suspect that my ethics committee will give approval for genetic screening for inherited cancers. There are several reasons why I believe it should. Firstly, the patients in question have a huge amount of detailed information about the diseases concerned, and also information about the screening process to avoid these genetic defects. In light of that information, they have, as responsible sensible people with first-hand knowledge, decided that it is right for them to have preimplantation diagnosis. Secondly, we, as a country, have already agreed the principle which argues that full human life does not effectively begin at fertilisation. Few of us, for example, would doubt the right of these women to use a contraceptive coil which destroys early embryos, in order to prevent having a child at risk. Thirdly, I believe that ethics committees should at least take into account that the application has been made by health care professionals who have got to know and understand the problems of the patient concerned. The judgment of these doctors and nurses should not be underestimated; distant ethics committees have been known to make serious errors of judgment when they ignore the first-hand experience of those in the front line. Finally, they need to consider the autonomy of the patient, and weigh this against the interests of society which are actually very seldom jeopardised in taking decisions of this sort. To my mind, doctors should recognise that their first responsibility is nearly always to the individual patient, and only thereafter to society. Had Nazi doctors recognised this, they might not have made some of the immoral decisions that they did.

There is an alternative to embryo screening. It is gene therapy. Embryo screening involves the discarding and hence destruction of embryos affected with these serious disorders. Gene therapy means their treatment. Even vigorous political opponents of embryo research like Enoch Powell MP and Sir Bernard Braine MP, who were both implacably opposed to our work on embryos, argued in favour of treating the embryo.

I should point out that there are two types of gene therapy. The first, with which we are not concerned here, is somatic cell therapy. This involves inserting healthy genes into the body so that they will be incorporated into a particular tissue and there make the desired protein. A good example is the aerosol being developed for cystic fibrosis victims. When their lungs are damaged, they can inhale the gene which will hopefully become incorporated into the lung tissues sending instructions to the cells there to make the proteins missing in cystic fibrosis. The problem with somatic cell therapy is that it needs to be given after the disease has already manifested itself. Scar tissue will be likely to have set in, so somatic therapy generally cannot be a total cure. Because the gene is only incorporated into developed or developing target tissues, it has no effect on the germ cells, so no injected genes are passed on to the next generation.

Germ line gene therapy is the incorporation of needed genes into the embryo itself. An extremely fine pipette is used to inject a tiny fragment of DNA which becomes incorporated into the nucleus, and thereafter all cells in the embryo carry the gene, including the germ cells. Thus germ line therapy cures the particular disease in future generations. Preimplantation screening of embryos with transfer of unaffected embryos may eradicate the disease for some families, but not always. This depends on whether carrier embryos are transferred or not. With preimplantation diagnosis it is often necessary to transfer a carrier embryo to have the best chance of pregnancy. This is because, in a particular group of embryos screened, there may on occasions be no completely normal embryos present. A good example of this is seen with our embryo screening for sex-linked diseases such as haemophilia. If we transfer a female she will not be affected, but a female carrier may pass the disease on to one of her children. Thus it was with Queen Victoria and the Tsarina. They did not have haemophilia themselves, but many of their male descendants suffered with this disease.

There are powerful arguments in favour of germ line gene therapy. It is a moral obligation for doctors to offer the best treatment possible. Gene therapy treats the disease before it appears, and ensures that future generations will not suffer from it. It also protects the autonomy of parents who, being offered it as a possible therapy, have the option of a variety of choices from which to make a decision. It does not involve destroying the human embryo but rather protects its sanctity. It is also possibly likely to be the most effective treatment. One limitation of gene therapy for diseases such as cystic fibrosis is that by the time somatic cell gene therapy is started, scar tissue has already formed and there is some impairment of organ function. So it will not stop a child with established cystic fibrosis from being breathless on exertion or being prone to chest infection. Lastly, the implementation of germ line therapy will be immensely important to scientific enquiry. By its study there is no doubt we would understand much more about how genes enter the embryonic cells and how their expression is controlled. We would gain information of immense importance to human genetics.

Against germ line gene therapy is the fact that it is likely to be a relatively expensive treatment with only a limited application; expensive, for it involves access to the early human embryo, and limited because it could only be employed when one knew which gene was deficient and needed to be replaced in the embryonic cells. Thus it could only be of value for those families where there already was known to be a specific gene defect. Germ line therapy may not be safe either. Make a mistake with the gene that is incorporated, and that mistake is visited upon all future generations. Discarding an embryo or offering somatic gene therapy can only affect the embryo that is discarded, or the sick person who is undergoing the treatment. Moreover, any mistake would be irreversible; there is no doubt at all that mistakes would be made. Finally, germ line therapy may be seen to be the commencement of a slippery slope.

The most obvious slippery slope argument is that, given time, parents will not only want to prevent severe defects, but later less serious ones. From thence it would seem it would be a small step to actually enhance certain characteristics and produce so-called 'designer babies'. Once we have the technology, influential and wealthy parents will invoke the genetic fairy godmother, who will endow the little prince with intelligence, strength, beauty, fortitude, as well as ensuring that it will not develop diabetes. It could be that from there it is another small step for totalitarian governments to genetically engineer certain desirable traits which would further the ends of the state, such as height, aggression and limited intelligence. To prevent this, it is said, all germ line modification should be banned.

Like all slippery slope arguments, none of this to my mind makes a great deal of sense. Robertson, in his interesting book *Children of Choice: Freedom and the new Reproductive Technologies*, points out that first of all there is by no means any certainty that the predictions at the end of the slippery slope will definitely happen. Secondly, he says that the feared extension of such work may not be so undesirable as expected. Thirdly, there may be ways of limiting the undesirable uses, whilst promoting the good uses. It is this last argument with which I have very great sympathy. I do not believe that humans have ever really banned a technology simply because it is harmful. We have the motor car which does immense damage to our environment. We have the electronics industry which is so effective at making sophisticated weaponry. We have aircraft which can be used to obliterate populations many thousands of feet below them. But we do not, and should not, ban these technologies. Rather we should control them and use the the good that they undoubtedly bring mankind. If we were to ban gene therapy, we would have to show that probability of future harm outweighed its individual benefits. Simply to ban it on any other basis would be arbitrary.

But my main criticism of germ line gene therapy is primarily a practical one. In order for gene therapy to work at all, any gene that is therapeutically inserted into the embryo must function normally, providing its usual message to the cell, and fully. There would also need to be assurance that the gene was incorporated in the DNA string at the right point. Failure to do so could have serious and unpredictable effects. Next, there must be no risk of causing mutations which might affect the individual. It would, for example, be stupid to cure cystic fibrosis only to find that the 'cured' person has developed leukaemia. Nor should there be any genetic side-effects, or long-term effects. The cystic fibrosis might be cured, but other genes then cease to function. Alternatively, the inserted gene might work for the first year or two of life and then stop expressing. Another problem to overcome would be that there should be no risk of lethal damage to the embryo. One of the reasons in favour of germ line therapy is that it acknowledges a basic respect for the embryo which is considered worthy of treatment. To kill as a result of the procedure would hardly be very desirable. Moreover, the embryo must not only survive the gene injection, it must be capable of implantation into the uterus afterwards, with normal growth during pregnancy. Lastly, there must be no lingering problem from the original gene defect.

These criteria are a pretty tall order. Obviously there is no precedent for what happens in humans because at the moment gene therapy in the human embryo is banned. The medical research funding organisations from the developed countries met in Europe a few years ago and called for a moratorium. This has been strictly observed, even though for most of the time since their declaration there has been no formal legislation in almost any country forbidding it, except Germany and the UK. We do, however, have information from other mammals, notably the mouse which is the common animal genetic model.

A number of scientists have developed transgenic mice which act as an important model for human disease. There are a number of laboratories around the world which specialise in making transgenics. A specific gene, thought to be the cause of a particular human disease, is injected into the mouse embryo before implantation, the embryo is transferred back into the uterus, and if it develops and is delivered, the effects of the gene may be studied and possibly various therapies used experimentally to see what beneficial effect they have. One such laboratory, in California, is run by Dr Carol

Readhead, who has great expertise in this area. Amongst other advances, she has produced transgenic mice who have a problem with myelin production, and these mice, although not particularly ill, make an important model for multiple sclerosis – sadly a progressive, paralysing condition which is common in humans. I recently asked her how effective her attempts at incorporating a given gene are.

Germ line gene insertion, it turns out, is highly inefficient. It is also very dangerous for the embryo. Typically, after any gene is inserted a significant number of mouse embryos invariably die. The insertion itself is lethal for them. Moreover, about 20% more embryos do not implant than would be expected after the transfer of normal mice embryos. On average, in the survivors, the gene only is incorporated into the DNA in at most 30% of the remaining animals. When the gene does express (or work), it usually only expresses at about 50% of full activity and this always varies. Moreover, the level of expression may initially be high but often gradually falls away after some months. Lastly, in a few of the surviving mice there are mutagenic effects. Many years ago, I remember paying a visit to Jon Gordon's laboratory in New York. He was one of the first experimenters to make transgenics. When I saw his mice who had had, for example, bone marrow genes inserted, it was disturbing to see how many had quite unrelated abnormalities of the tail, the eyes and the fur. Although most of those problems have now been largely solved, there still is a risk.

Imagine all this translated into the human. Leaving aside the number of embryos which would die or not implant and thus make the process extremely inefficient, there is the extraordinary unpredictability of everything if a viable pregnancy does form. The cystic fibrosis might be cured consistently in a minor proportion of cases or it might just be less severe. There could be a risk of the full disease returning after a few years. Moreover, there might be other essential genes which now no longer work, even though the cystic fibrosis is cured. But above all there is the awful concern of causing a severe abnormality in the baby, which would be completely unpredictable. I cannot imagine any doctor taking the risk of such an abnormality happening. Leaving aside any moral responsibility, the medico-legal risk would be prohibitive.

It would surely be very much easier simply to discard our embryo with cystic fibrosis. Before we did the gene therapy, we would need to make our preimplantation diagnosis in any case. There would be no point at all in inserting a gene into an embryo which did not need it. For all these reasons I suspect there may be a much rosier future for screening than for therapy.

If I am wrong and gene therapy does go ahead, what about those desirable characteristics given as a result of 'genetic enhancement'? Why not insert just a little more intellectual ability? In spite of the moral indignation which is usually expressed when this subject is discussed amongst the great and the good, there is, I believe, no definite right answer to this question. If we really are to value the next generation, what is essentially wrong in giving one's children every possible advantage in life? We parents now manipulate traits in our children in all sorts of social and educational ways. These include extra trumpet lessons for the musical child, regular extra-curricular lessons in arithmetic for the entrant to a particular school, and tennis and football courses at sports clubs. Although drugs are banned to improve athletic performance (though one might observe it is hard to say why the administration of a completely harmless drug is intrinsically wrong in such circum-stances), we certainly approve of orthodontic treatment to improve physical beauty. If a child is short in stature, we consider giving growth hormone, whether or not there is a specific disease process involved. No right-minded person that I know of objects to fluoride toothpaste or to regular doses of vitamins, even in children having a perfectly healthy diet.

Of course, all the above actions may increase class or racial prejudice. They may increase the social gap between rich and poor. They may encourage people to regard children as a commodity in certain circumstances. They may simply give some children advantages over others. But the fact of the matter remains that in our society we allow parents considerable latitude and discretion in their nurture of children. With the irrational exception of physique-enhancing drugs, nobody has seriously suggested a constitutionally imposed ban.

So what is wrong with prenatal enhancement of desirable characteristics? Possibly the first consideration is that genetically induced characteristics may in some way have a more powerful effect than those induced by environment after birth. There is no evidence for this one way or the other at present. Other people see enhancing desirable characteristics as violating religious values, in not accepting what God has given us. Yet, a few years ago, the last Chief Rabbi, Lord Jakobovits who is undoubtedly a much respected religious leader, became embroiled when he stated in a letter to *The Times* that if it were possible to genetically engineer the gene for homosexuality out of individuals, it would be perfectly moral and religiously acceptable to do so. Lord Jakobovits came under attack from a number of homosexual groups, but no serious religious objections were made to his notion that it would be morally proper to 'enhance' a person's genetic heritage. Sadly, because his opinion involved questions regarding the nature of homosexuality, his views were not seriously discussed or considered. Perhaps the main consideration is the fact that genetic enhancement could be harmful to children. Even assuming that the technical and chemical problems of gene expression and gene insertion were made completely safe, there is still the worry that there could be severe psychological problems for children. For example, they might not reach up to their parents' expectations or the investment value that their parents felt they should have. There certainly could be a serious threat to a child's self-esteem, or possibly to his view of others who were not so fortunately endowed by their parents.

There is another concern which is well illustrated by the argument which erupted over the 'homosexual gene'. What we regard as desirable or undesirable characteristics are made subjectively in the narrow understanding of our values and our society. If we engineer 'desirable' characteristics genetically, not only would we be committing our children to our concept of beauty, for example, but their children and all future generations. Generations to come would be condemned to a being which we had forced upon them, using a sense of values and judgments which are doubtful in our society, and could be damaging or worse in theirs.

None of these arguments seems to be an overwhelming case for a halt on genetic engineering. Whilst the term has an extremely negative connotation, reflection suggests that genetic enhancement might simply imply another example of the many inequalities which are inherent in human society.

However, I do not consider that genetic engineering is at all feasible now or in the mid-term future. Let us, for a moment, consider diabetes mellitus. Diabetes is an extraordinarily well-defined disease. It is caused by our pancreas being no longer able to produce the protein insulin. This results in the disorganisation of sugar metabolism, with all the side-effects which can occur as a result of having a high blood sugar. But the high blood sugar, and the effects on the heart, arteries, kidneys, brain, eyes, and nervous system are not primarily a genetic result. The genetic defect simply causes the pancreatic failure and the lack of insulin. Diabetes is technically a very well defined phenotype. The phenotype is the specific bodily expression of the genetic influence. Yet, the case of diabetes is like strength or beauty. It is polygenic – the interaction of many different genes. Remarkably, at least 23 have been incriminated, on no fewer than 17 different chromosome pairs. So here we have a really straightforward characteristic – no insulin produced by the pancreas – yet there is a wide range of different completely unrelated genes potentially associated with it. Consequently it would seem extremely unlikely that there could be a serious genetic cure for most cases of this disease in the reasonable future. If we have difficulty over detecting one very specific defect like Lesch-Nyhan syndrome (page 126), a real genetic cure for diabetes would seem very remote. But diabetes is well defined. How can we define beauty – or intelligence? I think the practical problems are so great that, for a long time at least, the human genome is safe in our hands.

There is another concern that I have about genetic engineering. A species is defined essentially by its genetic structure. A dog is not a dog simply because it has four legs, a tail, whiskers, and teeth which chew meat. So has a cat. The phenotype or appearance and structure of an animal may give clues to how species are related genetically, but it is the genotype or specific genetic structure which defines a species. One of the strongest pieces of evidence in favour of the theory of evolution is based on similarities in the DNA. True that Darwin arrived at his theory by examining the phenotype, but it is really the development of modern genetics which has provided the irrefutable, overwhelming evidence. We are close to the chimpanzee, not because the chimp looks human, or even because his brain is closest to our own, but because our DNA shows strong evidence of our having evolved from the same stock. This DNA has slowly been modified over hundreds of thousands of years. Randomly produced new mutations, slight changes in the DNA, have resulted in a modified phenotype or characteristics. When those characteristics have favoured survival, breeding amongst those that have survived have led to that particular genome continuing. This is the basis for survival of the fittest.

It is interesting to consider whether evolution ends with Man. Perhaps it truly does. Man may be the pinnacle of divine achievement because natural evolution will go no further. Perhaps it is not too arrogant to suggest that man has reached the state where, with his highly developed brain and with his ability to use tools, he has the means to manipulate his own environment. Survival of the fittest now becomes less likely to be needed biologically because mankind will develop the ability to protect itself against natural onslaught. The future would seem therefore to be either total destruction of man due to monstrous calamity, or survival more or less in our present form.

The curiosity of human genetic engineering is that, by tampering with our own DNA, we could actually change or hasten the process of evolution, producing new species. If we did this with the human genome, we could in a short time, produce a humanly derived species which in fact is no longer human. This concept is startling, but it seems to me to be a logical result of genetic engineering. It undermines our basic concept of human life and its sanctity. We regard human life as sacred. Human life is sacred and subject to ultimate protection because we humans are made in the image of God. We might destroy God's work from time to time and this may be seen as undesirable. However, it is absolute that we do not destroy His very image. We may only do that on rare occasions when the aim is to protect other human life, as we see it for the greater good of humanity.

When doctors like myself work on genetics or embryos, we do so with the ultimate goal of preserving and maintaining human life. It has been said, pejoratively, that those creating human embryos are creating life. The accusation is that we are attempting to supplant God, by meddling with His Creation. This is wrong. We are not creating life at all, but making it. The difference is simple – to 'create' means essentially to derive something from nothing. That is the divine prerogative. When, however, we merely 'make' something, we are using the material already available, the materials of Creation, deriving something from something else. So making embryos in the test tube is not supplanting God, but rather imitating Him – the Jewish concept is 'walking in His ways' or 'imitatio Dei' which is one of the ultimate goals of mankind.

So the challenging question is this. If we genetically engineer a new being – say a 'superhuman', is this an act of creation? Probably not, because we are still using God's materials. Is this 'superhuman' made in God's image? Presumably not, and by making him perhaps we would be attempting to supplant God, rather than merely imitate Him. At this stage human life would no longer be sacred.

At his creation, the first divine command to Man in the Bible is, 'Be fruitful and multiply, and replenish the earth and subdue it' (Genesis I: 28). We have certainly been fruitful as a species, and we continue to multiply. It is less clear whether we have replenished the earth. One serious criticism of our work that is continually heard concerns the wisdom and ethicality of promoting fertility when the world's population is increasing so dramatically. The number of humans on the planet increases by about 10,000 each hour – about 100 million annually. The human species has been on earth for about 200,000 years. In that time it grew from nothing to around 2 billion by 1932, when the first moderately accurate estimate of population was made. Since then it more than doubled by 1989, reaching 5.2 billion. It is expected that there will be 7 billion humans in fifteen years' time. Growth rates are fastest in countries that can least afford it, whilst in Europe and North America, population growth is virtually at a standstill. We, in the rich countries are becoming increasingly outnumbered. However, the biological problems which face humanity as a consequence of burgeoning world population are actually universal. In the industrialised countries the issues are pollution, particularly of both fresh and sea water and air (we have already seen how this may cause a decrease in male fertility), lack of space in our cities and in the countryside and contaminated foods. Overfishing makes it probable, according to a recent report, that most edible sea fish will be extinct in the next ten to fifteen years, and we shall be reduced to fish farming. In the developing world, pollution is also a serious problem and the economic pressures there make its control much more problematic. Overpopulation brings with it disease and famine, which follows loss of farming land and good soil, deforestation which threatens the climate, social instability and occasionally civil war. In the countries where poverty is most marked, there is a direct relationship between this and inadequate unpopulated land. This ironically increases the need to produce children in those populations, as the high infant mortality rate and the death of young people from disease, requires parents to continue to procreate for children to provide for their old age.

Rich countries are a greater threat to the ecology, partly because they consume far more of the world's resources per capita, and partly because they control so many of the resources and the natural materials. This affluence and the increasing industrialisation of our society is leading to climatic changes, whose effects may further damage the environment in which we live.

Added to all this, medicine is improving in such a way that in the advanced countries, people are now living to an unprecedented age. Before the seventeenth century, most people did not live much beyond forty. Before the beginning of this century, few people indeed lived longer than seventy-five years. Now half of the population of the USA and the UK will be expected to live longer than this, and one-quarter to the age of eighty-five. This aging population inevitably will consume more resources, particularly the medical support to control cancer, heart disease, skeletal diseases and all the other illnesses to which older people are far more prone.

Here, then, is a monstrous irony for such an infertile mammal. Whilst we value heritage and human continuity and apparently place great emphasis on the need for children, we are almost completely failing to come up with solutions to what is probably the most serious problem facing the planet. In a real sense, we have deprived our children of a good environment. We have taken from them, almost certainly irreversibly, some of the planet's productivity and are bequeathing them an increasingly hostile milieu.

Of course this does not mean that the human species will die out. But it is likely that, unless we control things effectively and halt the damage we are doing, the planet will take steps to control us. Comfortable human existence, as we see it in the western world, is indeed under judgment and we need to be much more thoughtful about these issues before a cataclysm hits our children.

There are two different ways in which a commitment to an understanding of reproductive technology can help alleviate the mess which is threatening us. Firstly, it must not be forgotten that reproductive research is as much about control of fertility as it is about its promotion. There are indications that if we can improve the lot of those in the developing world and halt their poverty and ameliorate disease, the advances in contraception that our work can bring will be of immense importance. Let me give just one example. With access to the human embryo, produced as a result of IVF techniques, we can look at the surface of the embryo and also of the eggs and sperm that preceded its development. Results of the examination of those proteins may provide the new generation of contraceptives. It is probable that, by the end of the decade, we may have much safer and more acceptable ways to limit fertility by providing simple vaccines which produce an immune reaction against those proteins. Alternatively, methods for vaccination against the early pregnancy hormone, which is itself a protein, or possibly against placental cells, may become effective and very acceptable when they are developed. These methods need IVF and access to the embryo for their research and development. This is because it is necessary to ensure that the vaccines do not cause embryonic or fetal abnormalities in the event of contraceptive failure. We also have to ensure that the vaccines are reversible, and that they can have no long-term effect on any baby that is born to a previously vaccinated mother, such as unwanted depression of its fertility.

Reproductive technology is of growing importance for another reason. Both the technology itself and the increasing debate about its uses, have unquestionably heightened public awareness of what having and not having children means to us. The debate has repeatedly emphasised our collective reproductive responsibilities, not just to our own nuclear family but in more global terms too. It is remarkable how many developed and developing countries now emphasise the need for reproductive medicine. In the last three years, I have attended national conferences on IVF in seven developing world countries. It seems surprising that these countries hold conferences on IVF at all when, after all, infertility would not appear to be much of a problem. The threat that these countries face is the threat to their society that overpopulation brings. They see this vividly every day as they walk the streets; to us the sight of people giving birth, feeding and dying on the same piece of pavement is just the briefest image on a television screen. Yet what was impressive about all these conferences was that, unlike similar conferences on the same theme in this country, all were invariably attended by the minister of health of that country. Frequently ministers or senior officials, would make important speeches, or join debates about the repro- ductive technologies. What is most encouraging is that in the countries that I have visited in this capacity, the level of these debates and discussions has been of an increasingly high standard with much thought given to the subject matter.

This is surely the message with regard to resources. Our role as scientists and doctors developing techniques like IVF must always be to recognise the responsibility we have towards the next generation. There are no longer national boundaries. What will affect our children will be as much global as local. As we help make these technologies increasingly available we have to remember why we are doing this work.

IVF techniques hold not only promise, but also risks. There is a close ethical parallel which was repeatedly drawn by thinkers in the sixteenth century, when alchemists were trying to find the elixir of life or attempting to transmute base metals into gold. Some of them subsumed everything, including their moral feelings, in the futile pursuit of a technology which ultimately could not benefit society. Peter Brueghel the Elder drew an elegant woodcut (1555) now in the Künst Museum in Berlin, 'Alghemiste', depicting the alchemist neglecting his family, the next generation, in frivolous technological endeavours. He sits to one side at his desk, reading from his huge tome and directing operations in his laboratory. His two oblivious technicians, hats over their eyes, are totally intent on their crucibles and tripods. His children run amok in the cupboard, one with the coal skuttle over his head. In the centre of the picture sits his wife, with all resources consumed, holding an empty purse. Through the window of the laboratory we see the future – his children are being conducted to the poor house. The word 'Alghemiste' is a pun in Flemish. It means, of course, 'Alchemist'. But it also means 'All is lost' or perhaps more poignantly still 'All has miscarried'. It is incumbent on us as scientists and clinicians to ensure that this intriguing and complex work does not produce human miscarriage, but that it is ultimately used for human good and the promotion of the next generation.

Glossary

Adrenoleucodystrophy:
A disease which in certain form only affects boys. It causes spastic changes, mental deterioration, a kind of multiple sclerosis-like illness, and death, at the latest, by adolescence.

Amniocentesis:
A method for detecting abnormalities of the baby during pregnancy. Samples of fluid are drawn off using a fine needle inserted into the womb and analysed for chromosome or chemical abnormalities. A common method for diagnosing Down's syndrome.

Biopsy:
Taking a small piece of an organ or an embryo for analysis.

Buserelin:
Drug used to reduce the activity of the pituitary gland in the brain. Often administered by sniffing. Its use for two or three weeks prevents the ovary from producing its own follicles or hormones without external stimulation by fertility drugs. The effect is reversible within hours of stopping Buserelin.

Chromosomes:
The paired structures on which the genes are located. One of the pairs is inherited from the father, the other from the mother. Each human cell contains twenty-three pairs of chromosomes.

Chorion villus sampling:
Another method of detecting abnormalities of the baby during pregnancy. Can be done a bit earlier in pregnancy than amniocentesis but, because it involves taking cells from the developing placenta (or 'afterbirth'), it carries a slightly increased risk of miscarriage.

Clomiphene:
The fertility pill, normally called Clomid; taken to help ovulation.

Cystic fibrosis:
An inherited disorder which affects roughly one in 1600 individuals in the population. It causes severe damage and digestive problems. Sufferers are often underweight and have frequent severe chest infections.

Down's syndrome:
Caused by three copies (instead of a pair) of chromosome 21. Sometimes referred to as 'Mongolism'; causes mental retardation.

DI (Donor Insemination):
Use of a third party's sperm to generate a pregnancy. Insemination is usually done artificially into the vagina, but IVF may also be used.

Duchenne muscular dystrophy:
A fatal genetic defect. It is sex-linked, affecting only boys. Causes progressive muscle-wasting, necessitating life in a wheelchair.

Ectopic pregnancy:
Pregnancy outside the uterus – usually in the fallopian tube – which can occur in any woman with tubal damage, even after IVF.

Endocrinology:
The study of hormones and their regulation in the body.

Endometrium:
The lining of the womb, shed during menstruation.

Endometriosis:
Abnormal deposits of womb lining outside the womb, usually in organs nearby. Causes some internal bleeding and pain is common, particularly during periods.

Eugenics:
Literally means well born. Used by Francis Galton as a term coined to typify his 'judicious matings'. Reached its ultimate in Nazi Germany.

Fibroid:
Benign tumour of the uterus.

FSH:
Hormone produced by the pituitary gland, causing the ovary to produce follicles and eggs.

Genome:
The structure of the complete DNA in a species. The Human Genome Project is a multimillion dollar project designed to sequence the whole of the human genome by the beginning of the next century.

Germ line gene therapy:
Introducing new genes into a sperm, egg or embryo with the idea of curing a genetic defect. Because this has been introduced into a germ cell, the defect will be cured in future generations engendered from that germ line.

GIFT
The treatment by which eggs are removed from the ovary and mixed with sperm and then returned to one or other fallopian tube before fertilisation. Generally not as successful as IVF in the best clinics.

HCG:
Human chorionic gonadotrophin; a hormone which mimics the action of LH (see below), encouraging the ovary to develop follicles to ovulate.

HFEA:
Government regulatory body set up in 1990 to ensure proper IVF standards and to oversee research on the embryo. It was also empowered to regulate donor insemination.

Humegon:
Drug given by injection containing FSH (see opposite), which helps the ovary produce eggs.

Hydrosalpinx:
Water on the fallopian tube, usually caused by damage and blockage of the tube end by the ovary.

Hyperstimulation:
Overvigorous response of the ovary to fertility drugs, causing swelling of the ovary and discomfort.

Hysteroscopy:
Telescope inspection of the inside of the womb cavity.

ICSI:
Sperm injection directly into the egg to assist fertilisation.

IUI:
Intrauterine insemination; freshly produced semen is washed and filtered in the laboratory and then immediately injected into the uterine cavity. Cheaper than IVF but not as successful.

Immotile:
Not moving. Term applied frequently to damaged sperm.

Laparoscopy:
Telescope inspection of the pelvic organs and outside of the uterus.

Lesch-Nyhan syndrome:
An inherited sex-linked disorder affecting boys only. They suffer severe spasticity and mutilate themselves. It is caused by a private mutation in the DNA (qv).

LH:
The hormone from the pituitary gland which produces ovulation.

Microinjection:
Sperm injection (see ICSI).

PCR:
A diagnostic method for multiplying copy of the DNA until there is enough DNA to measure by molecular weight.

Percoll:
A slightly viscous fluid helpful in the laboratory for filtering the best sperm for some cases of male infertility.

Pergonal:
Drug given by injection containing FSH, which helps the ovary produce eggs. Similar to Humegon.

Pentoxyfylline:
Drug which when mixed with sperm sometimes increases their motility.

Phenotype:
The physical appearance and structure of a species or animal.

Pituitary gland:
The master gland at the base of the brain which controls many other glands in the body.

Polycystic ovary syndrome:
Common cause of failure to ovulate, but may also be associated with poor-quality eggs when ovulation does occur. However, polycystic ovaries, as opposed to the syndrome, are a common variant seen in healthy women, who are usually normally fertile.

Polygenic:
A characteristic or disease caused by a number of different genes working together.

Preimplantation:
Before implantation of the embryo i.e. in the first five days or so after fertilisation.

Primitive streak:
The first change in morphological appearance of the embryo from simply being a round cellular ball. The streak will develop into the central nervous system.

Private mutation:
A change in the one region of the DNA leading to a specific genetic disease. The precise structural defect in the DNA will only be found in one related family.

Seminology:
Study of seminal fluid.

Somatic cell gene therapy:
Treating a genetically based disease by inserting healthy genes into a differentiated tissue. A good example would be gene replacement

into the lungs of a cystic fibrosis sufferer, or insertion of genes into the bone marrow which then makes normal blood cells in a person with a congenital anaemia, such as thalassaemia.

SPUC:
Society for the Protection of the Unborn Child.

Tay-Sachs:
An inherited disorder, affecting mostly Jews of whom about one in thirty carry the gene. Babies affected by it have severe neurological problems.

Transgenic:
An animal which has had its genetic structure changed by gene insertion and which passes this new structure onto its offspring.

Thalassaemia:
An inherited blood disorder causing very severe anaemia. It is most common in South-East Asia and Mediterranean countries.

Warnock Commission:
A government commission set up to enquire into issues related to IVF, donor insemination and other aspects of human reproductive treatment. Chaired by Mary Warnock.

Y Chromosome:
The chromosome which carries the male-determining gene.

Zona pellucida:
The 'shell' around the eggs of all mammals which is largely protective.

Zygote:
A fertilised egg.

Index